Necessary Steps : A Family's Journey

A family's struggle with adolescent addiction

by

Jane I Barsumian

© 2004 by Jane I Barsumian. All rights reserved.

No part of this book may be reproduced, stored in a retrieval system, or transmitted by any means, electronic, mechanical, photocopying, recording, or otherwise, without written permission from the author.

First published by AuthorHouse 04/07/04

ISBN: 1-4140-8038-7 (e-book)
ISBN: 1-4184-2099-9 (Paperback)

Printed in the United States of America
Bloomington, IN

This book is printed on acid free paper.

In memory of

Tom and Ranie Eby

INTRODUCTION

December 7, 1988. We are on our way to court. Dan and I, together in the car, each deeply involved in our own thoughts, are traveling on a country road. Our minds, however, are embarking on a mental journey which will take at least three years, if not the remainder of our lives.

Our twenty three year old son, Burt, is about to be brought before a judge for violating the terms of his probation.

How ironic that this is the day Pearl Harbor was bombed! I think of President Roosevelt's speech to congress which I have seen many times on film: "December 7th, 1941, a day which shall live in infamy," he began as he described the attack on our country."

I am feeling attacked- *totally besieged* by an invisible enemy!

I search desperately through my brain for some phrase which might bring me comfort. Suddenly, from some very ordinary Sunday in church comes a piece of scripture, something about "putting on the whole armor of God." I recall on that particular Sunday, a lay person explained to him the "whole armor of God" meant that, unlike *human* armor with its metal joints and hinges, God's armor had no cracks. In God's armor you were completely sealed and protected from harm. I had found this to be an interesting thought at the time. Now, however, it took on an immediacy and intensity which made me appreciate the practice of Sunday church-going in a whole new way!

As I envisioned Dan and myself totally encased in God's armor- not at all an easy thing to do- I realized I was battling total terror.

The thing I most feared for the past two years had occurred. Our son had violated the terms of his probation.

***

CHAPTER ONE

In June, 1987, we appeared to be a "happy family in transition." Our oldest child, daughter, Leanne, twenty six, had completed her first year as an ordained Lutheran minister. Her husband, Kyle, was minister of music in a brand new church. Son, Jon, twenty three, was finishing his first year in medical school, and Burt, eighteen, had completed his freshman year of college. We had celebrated three graduations the year before with a family trip to Disney World. If you had asked us, we would smugly have given you a "recipe" for raising children successfully. We thought we must surely be model parents as we soaked up the compliments of family, friends and acquaintances.

In truth, we were not as together as we *appeared* to be, nor even as thought we were. Few, if any, families are. In the days to come, I would find myself continually sifting through past events looking for clues, signs, and indications in an attempt to find the *cause* of what I could not explain. After beginning the recovery process, one learns of addiction: "You didn't *cause* it and you can't *cure* it." Nevertheless, it seems while there may not be *one* cause, it is important to understand the contributing factors. Moreover, *in order to survive*, it is vital to determine one's legitimate path through this maze.

That spring, we did have a concern about Burt's third semester grades. His college was on a trimester system, and the first two sets of grades were alarming. We chalked up the first set to "freshman jitters." We knew he was essentially bright. He had been in a Gifted Program in elementary school. Why had there been no improvement during the second term? We intended to wait and see what his final grades were. Then we would all sit down together, as we prided ourselves on doing, and decide as a family what Burt should do.

We had been concerned about Burt's behavior before. He seemed to have outgrown his exasperating habit of testing limits. He seemed calmer than he had been as a small child. He had become outgoing and agreeable. His grades had been quite good in high school. We knew the first year of college is often difficult for kids who are on their own for the first time in their lives.

It didn't take long after his arrival home that early June, before I sensed that something was wrong. I could not put my finger on it. It wasn't so much *what* he did as the *way he did it.* He seemed genuinely glad to see me; yet, he disappeared almost immediately. Dan was away on business. I invited Burt out for dinner. I fantasized an unhurried meal in a favorite restaurant where he would relate to me, his mother, everything about his first year of college. When he suddenly had to leave half way through dinner, I tried to be philosophical. "After all," I told myself, "he's not your little 'Burt, the Squirt' anymore. You have to let him have his social life."

Four nights after his arrival, I awakened at 3:30 AM to the sound of our car coming in the driveway. I hadn't realized he had left the house! Earlier that evening, he and a friend were laughing in his room as I went off to bed. They must have left quietly. When it became light, I noticed the front fender of the car was crushed. He explained to me he had hit a deer. Somehow, it didn't make sense. Later, he changed his story. He was trying to avoid a deer and hit a rock! Puzzled, I asked him to drive me to the road where this had occurred. I asked him to find the rock he had hit. We drove around for hours; we never found it.

Shortly after that a friend commented that the back windows of the car looked as though they had been splashed in beer.

"Someone was partying in this car," he divined. The feeling persisted within me that something was terribly amiss.

"Burt," I intoned, "I don't know what *really* happened last night, but I know it was something strange. I would *like* to believe your story, but I just *can't*." He just looked at me blankly.

A week later, Burt's college grades arrived in the mail. They were *shocking*. His total average for his first year in college was 1.44 out of a possible 4.0. An accompanying letter suggested he not return until he had proven that he could do better!

I began to notice small things: lights left on, doors left standing open. There were unexplained phone calls in the middle of the night from people I did not know, and an air about my child that confused me. He seemed to be politely holding me at arm's length. Was this about privacy or secrecy? I wasn't sure. He was never impolite. In fact, he seemed to go out of his way to be considerate and helpful. The rest of the time, even when he was around, he seemed absent.

Burt began his summer job which had been arranged before he had arrived home for the summer. He was working at a nearby fruit stand. We were pleased to see him working so hard. We would stop to make small purchases just to witness our son courteously waiting on customers! It wasn't difficult to balance his small acts of carelessness with what we observed of him "on the job."

There were his small gestures which made me feel appreciated by him. He would arrive home from somewhere and present his father or myself with a small treat. Sometimes, he would tape a stick of gum to the steering wheel of my car. Any initial unwelcome thoughts which arose in my mind were thus quelled. I would begin to think about articles I had read describing marijuana as a drug which could create forgetfulness in people. This is what I thought one night when I went outside to close his car door after dark. I just happened to see the interior light glowing. But when I thought of all the kids I had ever met who admitted to "smoking pot" or "weed," he never seemed to fit the profile. Those kids seemed to wear earrings, have strange haircuts, wear horrible tee shirts with skulls on them, and swear at their parents. Burt just didn't fit this description.

Furthermore, it was difficult for us to envision ourselves as the parents of a drug user. We were parents who always took an interest in our children's activities. We volunteered to serve on committees with the Boy Scouts and had served as leaders of our church youth group. It seemed to me we fairly knocked ourselves out being attentive to our kids' needs.

Both Dan and I had experienced the breakdown of our original families.

Dan's parents divorced when he was twelve. His mother, who had been a nurturing person, gradually became mentally ill. We do not know to this day if her illness was the cause or the effect of the divorce. It was a complex matter with his mother's family bitterly taking sides against his father. This unfortunately served to keep Dan's father, who loved him, at a distance. His mother's family with good intentions, maneuvered him into taking on the role of "man of the house." No one believed him when he described his mother's increasingly disturbed behavior. For six years, he did the best he could to finish growing up in a situation in which he experienced abandonment and the need to be super responsible while attempting to control his mother's behavior and minimize its destructive effects. At age eighteen, after one year of college during which he found it impossible to study due to his mother's constant verbal interruptions and sometimes physical harassment, he despaired. He left home to join the Air Force. Some members of the family later realized what he had suffered. To their credit, they apologized to him. They made their mistakes in ignorance, not malice.

I, too, was left by my father. He died suddenly when I was fourteen, leaving my thirty eight year old mother to raise three children. With my grandmother's help, she was able to return to college and receive a teaching degree. We missed my father greatly. Not only did we miss his physical presence in the home, but I was unaware how much I depended on him for providing me with the framework for my life.

My father had overcome many obstacles. He had been a victim of the Armenian deportations of 1915 - 1917. He arrived in this country from Turkey at the age of seventeen. His family had been fairly well-to-do in the "old country," but everything had been taken from them. He and his brothers and a sister were fostered by their uncle who had been in the United States for several years, an established and respected medical doctor. This man and his wife, with no children of their own, fed, clothed and educated my father and his siblings. This tremendous example of generosity has been a great influence in my life.

My father instilled within me a respect and thirst for knowledge and a desire to develop my talents and abilities. He was so grateful for the opportunities which this country offered to him and to his children. Sometimes, he expected a great deal from me. I was afraid to disappoint him. There are great benefits to such an upbringing; however, at times, this has been hard on me when I have just needed to be loved for myself, no matter how unaccomplished or incompetent I might be feeling!

Dan was seventeen and I, fifteen, when we met. We found each other attractive enough; however, I believe that we each had a great need to regain the families we had lost. We married when Dan was twenty two and I, barely twenty. Our first child, daughter, Leanne, was born very soon thereafter. As happens so frequently, our intentions were good; but, our "people skills" were not entirely up to the task. Old feelings of abandonment , fears of rejection, low self-esteem, unmet dependency needs and unfulfilled, unrealistic expectations all began to wreak havoc in our marriage.

Of course, this first occurred at about the same time we finally managed to get on our feet financially.

Many times over the years, either one of us could have walked away. Yet, for some reason, we didn't. We stayed together and struggled with the issues. We received a great deal of counseling. At one point we actually did separate for a period of four months. The separation could have led to a divorce; instead, we reconciled and realized that the separation had been growth-producing for both of us.

It is true that this was not an easy thing for our children to go through; however, I believe that the overall message they received was a positive one of overcoming obstacles and moving on.

We had moved quite frequently in the early years of our marriage, a total of thirteen times in twenty years! The longest we had been in one place was four years. During this time, we had experienced the separation and reconciliation. I had returned to school to receive a master's degree in education in the field of counseling. Dan had a successful stint at being a manager for a major corporation. Our life seemed fairly stable and fulfilling. However, Dan felt the need to move for greater career options. In 1978, we reluctantly left our stable home and our supportive community for new challenges.

Our oldest child, Leanne, had graduated from high school and left for college in the mid-west. Our older son, Jon, had three remaining years of high school. He didn't want to move; however, he had developed an interest in first aid and was soon involved with the volunteer rescue squad in the community.

Burt, on the other hand, was a different story. Some of the activities in which he had participated were not available to him in the new area. He had won ribbons on the diving team, but the team in the new area was not of the same quality. There was no "gifted and talented" program in the new elementary school, either. Perhaps eventually we would have been able to help him find a comfortable niche of his own, except for one things: we became overwhelmed by a morass of problems created by the building of a house!

Three years of exhausting legal actions revolving around a totally unrewarding law suit left us with a loss of about fifty thousand dollars, the money we had set aside for our children's college education, just when it was needed. We almost lost our sanity, too! As I sift for clues to Burt's behavior, I recognize that no matter how well-intentioned we were as parents, the time and energy which the house fiasco diverted away from Burt may have been a negative factor.

Many youngsters begin to experiment with drugs when they go through puberty in about seventh or eighth grade. While Burt experienced behavioral problems during this period- something I attributed to his needing attention from his parents- he didn't get involved with the drug scene, then. Perhaps the presence of his brother who was five years older and still at home kept him from straying too far. They always teased each other, but they loved each other very much and basically got along well if I stayed out of the way. When Jon went away to college in a different state, Burt was thirteen.

He had some friends his own age, but he spent hours at our new computer, playing games.He also invented his own solution for the Rubick Cube- a popular puzzle at that time. He seemed to be more of a "loner" than his brother or sister. Leanne and Jon had always had each other. When Leanne left, Jon had Burt. Burt must have felt lonely. I, myself, enjoy the company of people, and so I was relieved when, at the beginning of his senior year in high school, Burt began to spend time with some friends.

Once or twice, Dan and I had returned from a weekend away during his senior year. We sensed that something had taken place during our absence. We could never be sure. There was a strange smell- like burnt incense and small scraps of trash which were foreign to me.

My thoughts return to the present as we pull into the court house parking lot. I wonder if we'll get to see Burt before his appearance. We have not spoken to him since shortly after Thanksgiving Day.

Dan and I had gone to be with family in Pennsylvania for the holiday. We had picked up our daughter, her husband, and our one month old granddaughter, Caryn. We drove to Pensacola, Florida, to visit Jon, who was doing a medical school rotation at the naval hospital there. Burt had promised that he would come to see us on Thanksgiving Day morning. He never showed up. He didn't answer the phone when we called him at the friend's house where he had been living for the past two months. I cried all the way to

Pennsylvania. We did speak to him briefly from Florida, a very disjointed conversation.

When we returned home, there was a message on our answering machine with a request to call his probation officer. There was also a letter from Burt. I opened it slowly. Somehow, I was not surprised to read: "Mom and dad, I am writing to you from the county jail." He had been there for four days! It was a good thing that we were far away. As he told us later, "It would not have done any good to call you. I know you would not have bailed me out." I believe he might have asked us for bail if we *had* been available. Burt already knew that simply knowing his predicament would have created pressure on us.

Our absence saved *him* from silently making his plea for help and saved *us* from the suffering we would have experienced in saying, "No."

Necessary Steps : A Family's Journey

As we walk into the courthouse, we have to pass the "holding tank"- a small room where jail inmates await their court appearances. Through a small window in the door, I catch a brief glimpse of Burt. I am aware that I have no feelings, whatsoever. I am completely numb.

We sit quietly in the rear of the court room. Burt's "friend," a rumored drug dealer, and his girl friend, nod and smile ingratiatingly at us. I feel slightly ill. I need to distract myself. I do not *want* to feel. I have brought my knitting and I focus on the feel of the yarn turning in my fingers. It is somehow soothing. It is something within my control. I envision God's armor clamping down tightly in our corner of the court room.

Several people come before the judge. He is lecturing them. Suddenly, I cannot believe I am here. It seems *so* unreal. My mind begins to wander.

It is 1978. We have recently moved to New York State from Pennsylvania. We are visiting our former neighbors at their house. After our overnight stay, we returned home. Our neighbors phoned us, and very tactfully asked if our ten year old son could possibly have helped himself to some silver dollars which had been given to their son. They were specialty items, not ordinary coins. Recalling that Burt once tried, at the tender age of five, to sell me back an opal which he had earlier pried out of my ring, we reluctantly agreed it was, indeed, possible. We asked Burt about it, hoping that he would tell the truth. We had no way of knowing for certain. He denied ever seeing any silver dollars. I had never felt that this issue had been satisfactorily resolved. Even though our former neighbors were very gracious and understanding, I always sensed that they believed Burt to be the thief!

On a rainy day in July, 1987, nearly ten years later, we finally received our answer to this riddle.

We were driving home from a drug and alcohol rehabilitation center. Three weeks earlier, we had succeeded in manipulating Burt into the treatment we believed he needed. Unfortunately, at this point Burt was truly unable to see that he *needed* treatment. It is clear to me, now, he was not being stubborn or oppositional. He could not see it any better than *we* could see how wrong we were when we continued to allow him to drive our cars after unsatisfactorily explained accidents.

The ride home from the rehab was painful for all. Burt could see that we were furious. We had failed in our mission. We were desperate to control him. We told him that he would probably be going to jail since he had left rehab. It wasn't true, but he wasn't sure. However, the experience was not totally unproductive. We *were* about to learn what had actually happened the night of his first accident!

Burt and a friend had drunk a few beers that night and ingested some type of drug. They then went out to "spin wheelies" in our car! The accident had occurred as a result and, in their intoxicated state, they responded in a very strange fashion. Rather than return home with the damaged car, they decided to go for a swim at a nearby poolside restaurant. They found the pool empty. Somewhat disappointed and looking to amuse themselves further, they found a door to the back of the restaurant unlocked. They entered and helped themselves to a keg of beer and several bottles of wine.

The discovery of this theft is a story which shall come later. The results led to Burt's arraignment for third degree burglary- felony charges! Since he had no prior record and youthful offender status, we had attempted to pressure him into treatment with the threat that he might be imprisoned. We had enlisted the help of a lawyer and the assistant district attorney to convince him that he needed to prove that he was truly remorseful by entering a formal treatment center. Later, through the course of our own treatment, we learned if a person's "wall of denial" cannot be breached, it is not possible to remand them into rehabilitation and achieve lasting results.

Burt did not really believe we could put him into jail, but he wasn't sure. He began to promise all sorts of things. He agreed to go for family counseling, he swore he would not drink alcohol or do drugs if he could just live at home. He agreed to abide by our rules. Then, in an act of what appeared to be genuine contrition, he confessed to the theft of the silver dollars. He cried bitterly and told us how much he regretted having done this, because the neighbors had been so good to him. He had simply used the coins- collector's items- in a slot machine! Since Burt confessed to this crime and agreed to our demands, we made peace. For the next year and one half, it was an uneasy time which merely postponed disaster.

***

CHAPTER TWO

The bailiff is announcing: People of New York State against Burtis Wilson. I stare as our son is led into the court room with his feet shackled in chains and his wrists linked by handcuffs.

All the years flash by in one moment. I am aware of every time he got himself into some kind of trouble. It all blends together, and I am amazed at how *much* trouble that was!

When he was not quite two, he skittered up a ladder onto a second story roof. We were cleaning the spouts. I looked up to see a tiny red sneaker disappear over the edge onto the roof. I held my breath while Dan went up and coaxed him to sit down so he could be safely reached. He used to enjoy lunging at his dad. We both prayed he wouldn't decide to play the "lunge game." Both Dan and Burt made it safely down to the ground.

Burt never took naps as a toddler and would be hyperactive from seven in the morning until eleven o'clock at night. It was *impossible* to keep him his crib, in his room, or *even in the house*! He could open a regular "hook and eye" latch, so we installed special "snap" latches to keep him inside the house.

Before installing the "snap" latches, we would get phone calls from neighbors telling us that "our little boy" had once again climbed up and was dangling from our front window sill. (These are not the same neighbors whose silver dollars were stolen. If we had stayed in this neighborhood, the folks there would probably have placed all their valuables in a bank vault!)

Setting limits for Burt was an enormous challenge. He seemed to find a way out of any consequence or punishment we would give him. Nothing seemed to condition him onto the desired "path" on which we were attempting to guide him. It took all our energy just to keep him from always having his way. I remember observing to our friends that Burt was "like two and one half *normal* kids." "If he had been our first, he would have been our last," was a comment we often made. Puzzled about his enormous energy output, I asked his pediatrician, "Isn't there *some*thing you can give him to quiet him down?" The kind doctor jokingly replied, "No, but I can give *you* something..."

All of this occurred in 1969, before the concept of hyperactivity had been fully developed. Even then, I knew that Burt was different. However, I didn't know what this difference meant. Whether he was hyperactive due to a chemical imbalance, family dynamics or because of our first move to a new town when he was eighteen months old, I do not know. He was what is known as a "good baby"- relatively calm and manageable the first year of his life. Then, it seemed that a switch was suddenly pulled somewhere in his tiny nervous system.

It is worth noting that Burt was absolutely adorable! With curly, golden hair, big blue eyes, (our other children were brown-eyed like their mother), and a heart-melting smile, he looked like a little "kewpie" doll. Another neighbor had him pegged. He used to startle me by inquiring about my angel, "And how *is* 'hell on wheels,' today?"

When we lived in The Netherlands, Burt attended a Dutch nursery school for four year olds. He had begun to speak after we moved to Holland, and learned English and Dutch simultaneously. Sometimes, he mixed both languages in the same sentence. We dubbed this mixture "Nederengles" or "N'english"! Our Dutch neighbors remarked to us that he sounded like a native. Dutch is a difficult, guttural tongue to pronounce. But, unlike the rest of us, Burt had *no accent*. He fit in completely!

Returning to "the states," after an absence of two years, (*half* of Burt's short life), was a major adjustment for our family. Dan had traveled a great deal while in Holland, so it was not as great a change for him. The rest of us had to readapt. Leanne and Jon were very aware of this. We were also, once again, getting used to a new community, new schools, new neighbors. Burt, however, was not at an age where any of this could be discussed. Most of what he remembered at the age of four was of his life in Holland! Once, I lamented the fact that eventually, he would probably forget the Dutch language he had learned naturally. He still referred to milk as "mel-lek" and he called what you put into a camera "fil-um." I found it interesting that the words which were most similar in both languages were the ones he retained.

However, Burt informed me not to worry about him losing his Dutch words, "Fredericka" (our neighbor's child) will make some more for me," he confidently stated. When I bemoaned not being able to get on an airplane and visit our friends and neighbors in The Netherlands, Burt asked me why I was so sad.

"We can't go back there, honey. It's too far away." "No it's not," Burt comforted me, "You just get on an airplane and ffffffft- you're there!" That's when I fully realized that geographical locations on the globe are not *miles* away, they are merely *dollars* away!

Burt began public school in the United States at a kindergarten within walking distance of our home. His teacher was not a particularly empathetic person.

I became alarmed one day when he returned home from school about ten minutes early. "Oh," I said, surprised, "is school over already?" "I *think* so," was his totally unguarded reply. I checked with a friend of mine who was the school secretary and discovered that *he had been absent all morning!*

He had stayed in the woods behind our house for nearly two and one half hours, and I never would have known if he had not been "off" on his timing by *ten minutes.!*

I began to volunteer as a teacher aide a few days a week in order to observe what was taking place in Burt's classroom. His teacher was a rather regimented person who seemed oblivious to anything except making sure that order was maintained and the children did what they were told! She became irritated with them if their shoes were untied!

Shortly before the end of the school term, I was asked to come to the school for a meeting with the school psychologist, the teacher and the principal. Knowing what it could be like at times to be Burt's parent, I felt apprehensive. In 1974, I had not yet returned to graduate school in the area of counseling. I felt overwhelmed by these three "experts." They explained to me that Burt seemed immature and unready for first grade. He didn't participate very much and held back unless the teacher insisted he do something. However, his I. Q. tests showed above average intelligence.

They also noted that he could not seem to sit still and concentrate on a set task.

I agreed with them that he did seem to have a great deal of energy. I shared my earlier concerns about him. However, I had observed that Burt had unusual powers of concentration if given a project to work on which he enjoyed or which he selected. For example, he *loved* dinosaurs and could name and describe almost every one of them as depicted in a much loved book.

What he did *not* do well was to conform, especially in a classroom with a regimental teacher! It was obvious to me he would not be any easier for the school personnel to "socialize" than he had been for his parents.

The school officials were full of terms such as "learning disabled," "minimum brain dysfunction," and "attention deficit disorder." I was alarmed. But, I told them they were not even considering the effect of the massive adjustment he had just made in moving into what, for him, was a *totally new* culture!

While it was exhausting, it was probably fortunate that only eight months later, we moved *again*. My friend, the school secretary, waited a few months before sending his records to the new school.

When Burt began first grade the next fall, he chanced upon a very warm, nurturing first grade teacher. This also happened to be the year in which Dan and I were separated. I was feeling emotionally overwhelmed. I believe this teacher's ability to foster Burt's individuality in such a way as to gain his cooperation my have been pivotal in his life!

Burt managed extremely well in first and second grade. He was happy in his new surroundings. As the family came together again, we found resources in our new community. Around us was a supportive network consisting of church and school. Leanne became active in the church youth group, eventually becoming president. It is from this experience that her interest grew in becoming a pastor. Dan and Jon became active in the Boy Scouts, and I returned to graduate school. Our lives felt secure and purposeful to me.

By the time Burt was in third grade he was enjoying success on the local diving team. Some of his energy was finally focused. He also qualified for the new "gifted and talented program" which actually encouraged and reinforced his divergent thinking instead of discouraging and disparaging it. A clever child with Burt's energy would be seen as either a blessing or a curse, depending upon the perceiver. Gifted children are often seen as an unwelcome "problem," rather than a challenge. They are often viewed as a threat by an insecure teacher.

While Leanne and Jon seemed able to manage in most situations of their growing up years, Burt seemed to have some special needs. I do not know why this was so. I don't think anyone knows. Whereas the older two were more externally oriented and socialized easily, Burt seemed more internally determined. There was something within him that seemed difficult, perhaps impossible, to access from the outside-in. The only way he seemed open to change of any kind was if it were his idea. External attempts to force change upon him made him firmly oppositional.This stubbornness, we later learned, is a characteristic of addictive thinking.

I believe Burt would probably have had difficulties in any case; however, I now believe he needed formal structure to a greater degree than our other two children. Without it, he seemed to have no concept of his own limitations, his own boundaries. He seemed to lack the ability to distinguish between where he ended and others began. Much later, a certified alcoholism counselor who was treating Burt explained to me "the disease of chemical dependency begins long before one takes one's first drink or ingests one's first drug."

Many folks have suggested what, to me, is obvious: did having an older brother and sister who were achievers put pressure upon Burt to perform? My answer is "probably, yes." However, strangely enough, Leanne and Jon were *not* super intellectuals or even superior students in high school, at least not as measured by grades! But they each *did* have one thing- a *dream!*

Leanne decided in her second year of college that she wanted to be a minister. She felt called to become a Lutheran pastor. As I have explained to many people, this was more likely *in spite of*, rather than because of, her parents. Jon fell in love with medicine after one CPR course which he took in a church youth group. When he found out he needed top grades in college to be admitted into medical school, he worked hard and *got* them! I know that Burt has the same potential to achieve. When he knows what he really wants, he will get it. But, this will be possible only when he has found a way out of the silent, subtle slavery known as addiction.

Denial is such an insidious thing! It is not what most people believe it is. Folks who are in recovery from addictions say, "Denial is not a river in Egypt!" It is crucial to understand that in terms of dependencies, denial is not a conscious choice to refuse to believe that something is so. The active alcoholic or drug addict really believes that it is okay for him or her to drink "a little." The cocaine or heroin addict, the "weed smoker," or LSD. user, all believe they can manage their habits. The addicted gambler "knows" the next deal will be "the big one." The families of these folks honestly believe they are behaving in a healthy manner even as they lie, minimize and otherwise distort the truth, enabling their "identified patient" to avoid consequences, insisting all the while, that everything is fine.

A co-addict who is highly codependent upon the addict is, by definition, addicted to the addict. A system is created so that nothing changes. The addict is totally involved with the chosen drug or the behavior and the co-addict is totally involved with their own "drug of choice"- the addict!

At first, it did not seem possible that we could fit the model of an addictive family. Burt did not dress in a weird fashion and was very polite. His father was a hard worker and his mother was a psychotherapist who "knew all about people." We never saw Burt drunk from ingesting alcohol, and we were unaware of his being under the influence of other drugs while in our presence.

In his junior year of high school Burt's grades averaged an overall ninety two percent. One term his average was as high as ninety six! We were pleased because this is the year he would be sending transcripts to colleges. His college board scores totaled 1225, higher than those of either his brother or his sister. He applied to and was accepted by the same college from which his older brother had graduated. We were so pleased with Jon's experience; we were certain it would benefit Burt. Burt did not know what he wanted to do vocationally, but we reasoned that this was typical of most young people when they begin college.

Typical also, we thought, was the tendency to slacken off in the senior year. Later, we discovered that he was experimenting with marijuana and LSD, as well as drinking alcohol. However, all we experienced at the time was a young man beginning to bloom socially. He had a girl friend for the first time, and we liked her very much. There were other friends- bright, energetic young men and women. From all indications, Burt had everything that a contemporary young person could want: looks, intelligence, charm, and popularity. IN short, we thought, "he has it made!"

There was so much we did not know.

***

CHAPTER THREE

How did the social cancer of drug abuse metastasize to its current proportions? Since my youth in the early fifties and sixties, the increase in the problem of drug abuse and addiction is astronomical! Many parents do their best to provide children with care, concern, and quality time. They try to set firm boundaries. Yet, despite this, many of our young people simply implode.

I imagine it starts rather innocently- one or two beers, a joint. The celebrated peer group pressure- "everybody does it; don't be such a nerd." As adults, we enjoy our alcoholic beverages: our beer, cocktail hour and wine with dinner. For many of us it is not a problem. Thus, most of your youthful drinkers will quaff their brew puff their "weed" and be just fine years later.

Some will continue to overdo and become chronic abusers of chemicals, perhaps becoming physically addicted. *A certain group will become addicted from the very first drug use,* whether it is alcohol or some other substance. A combination of physical and psychological factors will determine the degree to which any individual will become a slave to substances and/or behaviors.

Scientists are just beginning to discover the underlying factors which cause or help to bring about the disease of addiction. I believe that someday, research will document that some individuals "win" a sort of genetic lottery. Congenital biochemistry will determine innate differences between those who are prone to addiction and those who are not. People who become addicts may be attempting to avoid emotional pain through self-medication. Feeling incomplete, they may be seeking simply to heal themselves. This is an entirely different way from how most of us view drug addicts!

Addiction is at root a spiritual concern because it represents a misdirected attempt to achieve wholeness, to experience inner completeness and satisfaction. We are all addicted to some extent. Some addictions are simply healthier than others.

All of us come into the world with wounds; they come from human birth, no matter what kind of family we grow up in, no matter what kind of society we live in. We long for a sense of completeness and wholeness and for an end to craving. Most often we look for satisfaction outside of ourselves. That is the root of addiction. Truly, whatever satisfaction we gain from food, drugs, sex, money, and other means of gratification, really comes from *inside* ourselves. We project our own power onto external substances and activities, allowing them to make us feel better temporarily. We give our power away in order to achieve a transient sense of wholeness, and then suffer because the objects we crave seem to have power over us.

Addiction can be cured only when we consciously experience this process, reclaim our power, and realize that wounds must be healed from within. Eventually, we may discover who we really are and identify with our true selves. Thus, the suffering and craving which comes from addictions has an emotional, psychological and spiritual component.

Biochemically, I am describing a condition similar to the disease of sugar diabetes where there is a lack of insulin hormone by which sugar is made able to be digested. While there is no *one* known physiological factor which causes the disease of chemical dependency, present research shows that a *combination* of genetic factors may predispose an individual to certain addictions.

I believe that our son, Burt, was predisposed to *immediate* addiction. We know that his great, great grandfather and one of his second cousins on the same side of the family both died at age forty seven of alcohol disease. For such a person as Burt to be part of that young crowd eager to experiment with what they see as "life's pleasures" meant to take an enormous risk with that young life. But none of us were aware of this!

A few weeks after Burt's accident with the car, Dan and I returned early from a weekend trip. The inside of the house was not markedly disturbed, but decorative articles had been moved around. In the kitchen, I noticed that someone had written strange phrases on a marker board. But when I looked out the sliding glass doors onto the back deck, I could see that the wrought iron table had been bent and all my little deck plants were missing. Almost in slow motion, I approached the deck rail. Thrown into the woods were kitchen utensils, miniature potted roses, beer cans, and plates. I was truly puzzled.

It was obvious from all of the empty beer cans that a party had taken place in our absence. About a year before, we had been away for a weekend. When we returned, I had the strange feeling something had taken place in our home while we were away. I could not find anything wrong, but the atmosphere seemed somehow disturbed. I do have a very sensitive nose which perhaps marginally detected some strange odors. At that time, we asked Burt if there had been anyone inside other than himself. Burt denied that anyone had been in the house. He did acknowledge "some kids tried to make me let them in." (How strange that we did not pursue this at the time...).

We explained then, under no circumstances should he invite or allow anyone to enter when we were away. We said if it ever happened to him again, he should call the police.

We told Burt since he had failed to call the police, we were now going to call them. If he could tell us the names of the trespassers, we would not call the police. We especially wanted to discover who had done all the damage! He flatly refused. "I'll pay for the damage and I'll clean up the mess," he volunteered, "but I *won't* give the names! So, we called the local police emergency dispatcher.

Burt was shocked and very angry. I imagine he was also frightened. And, so was I! For the first time ever, I began to get a glimpse of his hidden side- the side I would have recognized to be an addict.

What occurred next is, to me, a very unique and totally inexplicable phenomenon. I have my own ideas about it; however, it remains a mystery. While awaiting the arrival of the police, I experienced what I can only describe as an "inner voice,"- an inner "knowing." I was being "told" to go out into the woods. My sense was if I were to trust this intuition enough to act upon it, I would be led to something of significance. I had experienced such feelings in the past and they had always led to important results. Suspending my rational mind, I allowed myself to obey the impulse.

I felt rather stupid wandering into the woods without the slightest idea what I was doing there. Trusting in some greater good, I simply walked. The "knowing" led me to the ladder of Burt's tree house. "*Climb*," I intuited. I did not want to climb. I felt very silly, but I climbed, anyway. I felt myself mentally "split." There was a part of me watching and objecting to my illogical behavior, and a part of me totally in harmony with this strong, inner wish to comply.

At the top of the ladder, the next instruction came, "*Look!*" I looked into the tree house and *saw a huge keg of beer and numerous bottles of wine!* I was totally shocked, both at my discovery and, even more so, at the way in which I had made it. At that exact moment- *the police arrived.*

I could not possibly know at the time just how important this discovery was to be. As events unfolded, I came to believe a higher power intervened in our lives that day. My personal belief is this power is here in the world for all people and is made present to all in genuine need who believe and call upon it. To me, this is not a theoretical idea. The key is the word, *belief*-belief strong enough to be acted upon. I enflesh my belief in the person of Jesus of Nazareth. However, words are the development of humans, and therefore have limitations. The Almighty knows no bounds! I just know that the "Great I am" was *there* for *us!*

The eventual consequence of this discovery was to save our son from two kinds of death: spiritual and physical. Even if his physical body were to continue to exist, without recovery life would be meaningless. Tragically, many young people who become addicted end up in one of three conditions: physical death, incarceration or insanity.

The police were quite excited about my discovery. Later investigation revealed the beverages had been stolen from a local tavern. The owners had not even missed their stolen property!

At the time many of our friends thought the whole episode was blown totally out of proportion. They considered it to be a "college prank." We know now that if Burt had gotten away with this "prank," there would have been many more incidents of increasing severity. The inevitable painful consequences would have been far greater.

It was painful to see the encounter between Burt and the police. Burt was unbelievably rude and hostile. He showed such lack of respect for the local policemen, made nasty remarks, threatened and swore at them. I watched with tears streaming down my cheeks, nearly hysterical, as my charming, courteous son changed before my eyes into a raging demon! It was one of the most frightening scenes I have ever witnessed.

Until that moment, I had always been very skeptical of stories about demonic possession, but now, I began to wonder...

It took the local police one week to find the tavern from which the wine and beer had been stolen and to track down the nine people who had been to our house in our absence.

One Saturday afternoon, a young policeman whom we knew came to our house. He sat with us and very kindly projected the heart-rending journey upon which we were about to embark. "He's eighteen years old," he said, "and in this state he has Youthful Offender status. This means since this is his first offense, he will probably get probation. If he keeps himself out of trouble in the future, he won't have a criminal record. It will hopefully be a good learning experience for him." One more year and such an offense would generate a permanent criminal record.

Then the police officer told us something which astonished us. Every single one of the boys interviewed told the police that *Burt, himself, had been the person responsible for all the damage done!*

CHAPTER FOUR

There are many times when we do not get to choose what life brings to us. However, I have always felt that we *can* choose our *responses* to what comes. Later, when friends remarked that they didn't know how we ever managed to cope with our situation, I developed an unexpected reply: "Well, if given a choice between having a drug-addicted child or a trip to Bermuda, I would certainly have chosen the trip to Bermuda!" In reality, the *worst* part of this whole passage in our lives was *not* the knowledge that our son was addicted to drugs, it was *not knowing what the problem was!*

Much later, we were to learn Burt had invited the boys over that weekend. Some of them had been trying to prove who could hold the most liquor. They were also smoking marijuana. At one point Burt had consumed so much alcohol in a short period of time that he became in their words "wild.!" Some of the boys became frightened and left. The ones who stayed watched as he crashed porch furniture and threw plants, bottles and eating utensils into the woods. He didn't seem to know what he was doing. Significantly, he had no recollection of doing it. He was in a "black-out" from the ingestion of substances!

We were to learn in the future that experiencing "black-outs" very early in a drinking "career" is an early warning sign of addiction.

No one wants to come to the realization that their child has a drug problem. However, when you know something is very wrong and the "wrongness" has no name, it is even worse. More than anything else, we simply wanted some certainty. With awareness of the problem would come knowledge of what, if anything, could be done about it.

The police let us know their plan for Burt's arrest. They would pick him up at work at the fruit stand and take him into the station for a formal arraignment.

But first, he would be booked and finger-printed. They agreed to call us at a friend's home after making the arrest so we could come to be with him at the station.

We arrived to find a furious Burt! He would not even *look* at us. Nevertheless, we stood with him before the judge as he was arraigned on third degree burglary charges. He was released on his own recognizance. The local district attorney insisted crimes of this magnitude be handled by the county judge, not the local town justice. Since Burt had already admitted his guilt, there was no need for a trial. A court date was set for sentencing.

It was shortly before July 4th, 1987, not even one month since Burt's return home from college. It seemed like a year.

Although we had never seen Burt drunk or looking drugged, I believed this *must* be his problem. In fact, *I wanted it to be!* The only other options were criminality or insanity! "Here is where I can make a difference," I thought. With my knowledge of resources to aid in recovery from substance abuse I believed we might convince the district attorney to help us in using the threat of a possible jail sentence to intimidate Burt into a drug rehabilitation facility. I knew from my work the qualifications and locations of such places, and I was easily able to find one of them about an hour's drive away from our home. I phoned and made an appointment with a representative of Sycamore Park.

We visited the facility and had a tour of the beautiful buildings and grounds. It was difficult to believe this was a "rehab." Then we negotiated with the district attorney's officers. Burt's attorney whom we had hired despite Burt's objections, urged him to accept the offer. Very reluctantly, Burt agreed to a four week in-house treatment program at the drug rehabilitation facility I had found. We congratulated ourselves on a well-schemed plot to save our son from himself!

***

CHAPTER FIVE

On July 4, 1987, we drove to the rehabilitation facility to admit Burt into treatment for substance abuse. Due to the holiday, there was a "skeleton staff" on hand. He would spend the first twenty four to forty eight hours in "detox" where his body would be freed of any poisons. This is absolutely essential. Someone who has been using drugs consistently over a period of many weeks, months or years, could actually go into shock and die if suddenly taken off these substances! Burt would be closely watched. I did not believe his drug use had progressed to the point where he needed to be detoxified. I was right. He was in the earliest stage of addictive disease. While he felt drawn to use drugs, his body did not, yet, experience physical symptoms when he was not using. Therefore, one could say he was psychologically, but not physiologically addicted.

Unknown to us, the facility had chosen to place Burt, eighteen- a privotal age- in the adolescent treatment unit instead of the adult unit. Unfortunately, we had not been informed that the adolescent treatment program lasted *seven* weeks, not *four* like the adult program. We were to discover this fact on our way out the door!

We decided to say nothing of this to Burt who had agreed to a four week stay. We hoped he would eventually be open to whatever the experts thought necessary. We thought the treatment center could break through his "wall of denial." How little we really knew about addictive thinking!

During the first week in the treatment facility, he discovered his program lasted seven weeks. As his counselor explained to us, "he would have used *any* excuse to get what he wanted, which, as usual, was his *own* way, no matter the consequences." He simply did not, *could* not, have an awareness of the price he would pay! He had no concept of the pain we, his parents, were experiencing.

Necessary Steps : A Family's Journey

We were called by his counselor on a rainy day near the end of his fourth week of treatment. Burt wanted *out*. He had agreed to four weeks of treatment, *not* seven. He had nearly completed the fourth week. They had no right to hold him against his will if he chose to leave. We tried to convince ourselves that, if it had not been raining so hard, we would simply have left him there.

Before Burt left the rehab, his counselor sat down with him in front of us and literally predicted his future. She *knew*. She had made this same journey. We discovered an addict can fool anyone *except* another addict. She told him within the year, he would be using drugs so heavily he would totally lose control of himself. He would then be at risk of either overdosing or of engaging in criminal behavior. Her prediction varied from later reality only by the amount of time it took for him to "hit bottom." She predicted six months; he managed to limp through another one and one half years before bringing disaster upon himself to the point where he was forced to pay attention. We both hoped and feared that leaving treatment prematurely would bring about a jail term. However, since this was his very first offense, the actual sentence which he received for the third degree burglary was five years probation.

At the time, we were very distraught. We thought this attempt to intervene had been a failure because Burt left treatment. Now we realize he *did* learn valuable things about himself during this first stay in rehab- things which later would enable him to see himself more honestly.

My mind snaps to the present court room scene. I can hardly believe my eyes as I view my son in manacles- a mother's worst nightmare come true! "How does he see himself, now?" I wonder, as I stare at Burt. He looks fairly clean and neat in his T shirt and jeans. He is a nice-looking young man with an engaging smile. He is smiling, now, but with his mouth, only. His eyes look sad. He is trying to put forward his best self.

He has lost some weight. I am aware his body is still growing. Even at twenty, his hands and feet are slightly too large for his arms and legs. I desperately wish he were two years old again so I could just snatch him up in my arms and carry him away from all this. Somehow, I want to make everything right. Then I remember that even when he was two, I could not do it!

The judge is lecturing him. He deserves every word. This is a judge with a reputation for being tough. I do not want leniency. While I dread what is to come, I know it is absolutely necessary. Some children's characters seem to be easily molded and formed. They can be tapped into shape. Others seem to need to be clobbered with the proverbial "two-by-four." To people who do not suffer from addictions, the consequences an addict needs in order to realize his or her addiction must seem like overkill.

I clutch my "armor" tightly around me now. The judge is nearing the end of his sermon. He sentences

Burt to six months in the county jail with two months off "for good behavior." Burt will have to stay in jail for a minimum of four months! I hear a strange sound like the moan of a tiny, wounded animal. I realize it is coming from somewhere deep within me- the moan of a female human, a mother's cry.

***

CHAPTER SIX

For several days I simply lay on the living room couch. Every now and then, Dan would ask me if I wanted anything. I felt totally crushed. It was an effort to raise my hand. It was as though I were on a planet where gravity is five times that of earth. I was still trying to sort it out.

It had been one and one half years since Burt had left the drug rehabilitation center. At first, he was a model of decorum. We wrote a list of "house rules" by which we felt he could reasonably abide. The rules forbade the use of alcohol and other drugs. Burt was either to get a full-time job or take some courses at the local community college while working part-time. He was to pay a small fee for his room and board. Furthermore, he was to attend family therapy sessions.

Once again, we congratulated ourselves. We believe we had thought of everything! Dan and I wanted so much for this to work. If it did not, we felt strongly that we would have to ask him to leave. We also began to think perhaps his problem could be something other than drugs. He certainly didn't believe he had a drug problem! He seemed to need a lot of sleep. However, he was keeping very irregular hours, staying up most of the night and sleeping late into the day.

Burt got a job working the three to eleven shift at a nearby restaurant. We would go and have dinner there. He was a good waiter and was soon named "waiter of the month" with his photo displayed near the payment register. He charmed customers and co-workers with his courteous, helpful manner. For three or four days he seemed able to feel really well, leading what seemed to be a normal existence- sleeping at night and being awake and active during the day. From time to time, he would discuss possible plans to return to school after saving enough money. His plan was to work through the fall semester and return to his studies in January. We felt hopeful.

Burt's nineteenth birthday was the day before Halloween. Dan was away on a business trip, and I spent the weekend with friends at a nearby hunting cabin. I returned home to a message on our phone answering machine informing me that one of our cars had been found along a main road in town. It had been towed to a local garage. I felt my stomach clutch. I drove to the garage and found- no car! Then I drove to the restaurant to see Burt.

As I approached the restaurant parking lot, I again experienced an inexplicable "knowing." "That car has been in an accident," I was "told" from within. "Oh, *no*," countered my usual self, "Why would I think such a thing?" I turned into the lot. With relief I noticed the car appeared to be fine. "If you don't believe it," challenged the "voice" from within, "drive around to the other side of the car." The hair stood up on the back of my neck. I felt a chill. As I came around to the other side of the car, I was able to see that, sure enough, the entire right side of the car was bent in!

Burt was busily working. He seemed fine. He looked me in the eye and calmly explained he had been tuning the radio, was distracted, and ran off the road into the woods about a half mile from home. Again, I wanted so badly to believe him. I actually entertained the possibility that he was telling me the truth! I told him I didn't know *what* to believe, but I loved him and I was glad he hadn't been hurt.

Years later, we learned Burt had been under the influence of narcotics and alcohol when he passed out at the wheel and ran the car into the woods. Apparently, he was not injured and he managed to get himself home. He was not even aware the car had not accompanied him home! Since it was his birthday, his "druggy friends" had driven him around to various bars and night spots. One of them had asked Burt to drive him home. He has no recollection of doing any of this. The next morning, a couple friends stopped by. According to Burt, one of them awakened him with the question, "Hey, where'd you park the car?" Burt recalls his answer, "In the driveway." "No it's not," was the buddy's alarming reply.

"Oh my God," roared Burt as he bolted out of bed. He ran down the road, half-naked, a vague recollection of the night before emerging from the residue of chemicals in his brain. He ran the half mile to the spot where the car had left the road. *There was no car.* His first thought was that it had been stolen! Then, he observed the tire tracks in the mud and the broken branches where the car had gone into the woods. He figured it had probably been towed to a local garage.

Burt's buddies drove him to a local garage. There was our car- newly "decorated" on one side! He used eighty dollars of tip money to pay the towing fee and drove the car home. He was not aware the police had called and left a message on our answering machine.

Burt's mind- what a mixed blessing. He could create such terrible situations; yet, he was so clever at managing them! If it had not been for Burt's missing one small detail- the message- we would never had had first-hand knowledge of this particular accident. He probably would have told us he hit another deer!

It wasn't fun telling Dan the car needed body work. I could tell by his voice on the phone he resented being told about it. I resented always being alone when these accidents happened. We were both slowly being worn down. Living with a subtle drug addict is like being rubbed with very fine sand paper. You're not sure anything is actually happening; but, there is a fine residue of anxiety and a slight sense of your own diminishment. We experienced emotional erosion to the point where our whole family lost track of what is "normal." Dan and I began to blame each other for Burt's irresponsibility.

We told Burt he would have to pay to have the car repaired. However, our judgment had become warped. It astonishes us now that we continued to permit him to drive our cars. "After all," we reasoned, "he has to keep his job."

Because of his chronic tired feelings, we suggested to him that he might have a physical condition which needed attention. We set up an appointment with the family doctor. Unfortunately, it is not possible to test directly for a predisposition to addiction. The physical exam found him to be essentially healthy. We informed the physician of our concern. His opinion was, "If it looks like a duck, walks like a duck, and talks like a duck, it probably *is* a duck." The problem was in the early stages of addiction, there were only a *few* "duck-like" qualities in Burt. He wasn't "quacking" loud enough- *yet!*

***

CHAPTER SEVEN

Burt seemed to time any activity which could lead to a crisis to when his father was out of town. One night, very late before retiring, I stopped in to say good night to him. Something did not seem right. I walked over to his bed and touched- a pile of pillows and a football helmet all covered to resemble a sleeping form! "How many nights has he done *this* trick," I wondered.

I don't believe in searching through other people's possessions; however, under the circumstances, I decided it was time. It didn't take long. Right under his bed I found a box of small plastic wrappers, each containing a small quantity of marijuana. Obviously, it had been packaged for distribution.

The enormity of my discovery hit me bodily. I felt as though I had been physically beaten. My stomach quivered, my head pounded and my knees buckled. *While on probation for a felony offense, my son was dealing drugs!* I spent the night lying in bed staring at the ceiling feeling like hot needles were being poked into my brain. It was as though I had been attacked, nearly overwhelmed, by some force I could not understand. I did not know *how* to fight it. Nevertheless, once again, I would try.

Early the next morning after a sleepless night, my habit of trying to control the uncontrollable reasserted itself. Once again my addiction of attempting to control Burt's behavior only made things worse.

I *had* to get rid of those marijuana packets, not so he couldn't *smoke* them, but so he couldn't *sell* them! At first, I thought of taking them to a friend's home. But, *no*, that would endanger my friend. I thought of flushing them down the toilet or throwing them in the trash. However, I also intended to confront Burt with my discovery. (*I still* thought I could embarrass or intimidate him into good behavior!).

I seized upon the idea of hiding the packets by wrapping them in aluminum foil in the shape of a giant sandwich. I marked the package, "Sub" and placed it in the freezer. I remember feeling very clever and pleased with myself. I thought I had outwitted Burt. I experienced some relief from my feelings of helplessness.

Later that morning, Burt came home. We were about to interact, something we rarely did anymore. I heard him coming up the stairway from his room. Each step sounded ominous to me as though a Frankenstein or some other dreaded monster were approaching. When he spoke, his voice had an eerie, unfamiliar edge to it, "Mom, have you seen the box that was under my bed?"

Now it was my addiction which caused me to lie, "No," I answered as innocently as I could, "*What box?*" "Oh, I had a box there and it's gone." He didn't comment. The tone in his voice took on a hostile quality, "I think I know who has it and they're *not* going to get away with it!"

I had, indeed, outwitted Burt, but not in the way I intended. He returned to his room and emerged with what looked like weapons- two heavy sticks joined by a piece of rope! Suddenly, I realized that either he or someone else was going to get hurt. I had not considered this possibility. So, reluctantly, I confessed, "It was *me*, Burt, *I* took it."

Burt was obviously angry, but he remained very calm. He gazed steadily at me. "What did you do with the box?" Instead of embarrassing him, I had embarrassed myself. How had *I* become the villain? "Uh-uh- it's er...at a friend's," I muttered. "Where?" I gave him the name of the person I had first considered hiding it with. "I'm going over there and getting it," Burt stated. He frightened me. Who was inhabiting my son's body? Could this *possibly* be Burt?

Instead of feeling clever, I now felt totally powerless. While I didn't know it then, I know now I needed to fully experience my powerlessness over Burt in order to take the first step at overcoming my own addiction to attempting to control him.

"No," I said, fearfully, "it's not there; I lied." I could see he was not going to let me get away with my "crime."

What ensued was a struggle between mother and son. Yet, it was strangely muted. The only physical part was he would not allow me to leave the room. He never touched me; he simply blocked the doorway so I could not leave. All I could think of was how small he had once been and how large he was now! I cried, I yelled, I screamed, I got hysterical. The accumulated frustration of the past months totally took over and I became the one possessed!

"Either give me the box or pay me for it," he intoned ominously in a flat, unemotional voice. I realized I was close to a complete breakdown. I was in danger of escalating the crisis. I needed to restore calm in any way I could. All that was left for me to control was myself, and that I could barely manage to do. What were my options? Thoughts raced through my brain as I struggled with the storm of emotion which was threatening to engulf me. I decided we could work on resolving the situation later. If I threatened him or lost control and thrashed out physically, I would only make a bad situation worse.

I chose to allow myself to feel humiliated for the moment and wrote a check for three hundred and fifty dollars. *I now owned a quarter of a pound of marijuana!*

Although I had been offered marijuana once in the mid-seventies by a friend, I had made a considered decision *not* to try it. I was curious and very tempted.

Many people I knew had done it at least once. The fact that I had three children nearing adolescence gave me the motivation to "just say no." My rule of thumb for child-rearing included the idea that if I didn't want them to do something, I had better not do it, either.

"How ironic," I thought, "I'm buying drugs and my son is selling them to me!" Burt took the check and disappeared.

***

CHAPTER EIGHT

When Dan returned home from his business trip, he could see I was physically, mentally and emotionally exhausted. We decided to do something very healthy. We removed ourselves from the scene. We drove to Atlantic City to a time-share apartment for a week. Why Atlantic City? Why not? I had never been there. It really didn't matter *where* we went just so it was- *away*! The whole time we were driving, I thought people were following us. I had no idea just how involved Burt was in illegal activities. One could say I was paranoid; yet, I had reasons to believe people might be after us!

When we arrived in Atlantic City, we walked the boardwalk. We even went into some of the Casinos. I tried very hard to get my mind off of Burt. I experienced what I now understand as withdrawal symptoms. I went in and out of nausea and sleeplessness as I forced myself with great difficulty to focus on things other than attempts to control our uncontrollable son. Moreover, we took a huge step for ourselves- we attended our first Alanon meeting.

We had not once in all this time done the most obvious thing- gotten help for ourselves! This huge resistance is a phenomenon I had seen before and still see in others. Just as the addict refuses help, so does the co-dependent who is involved with the addict. Our denial had been as great as Burt's. We could not appreciate how a group of strangers with addicted relatives could possibly be of help. After all, we thought, *we* didn't have a problem! However, it had been suggested to us by professionals in the field of substance abuse treatment and it seemed to be the only thing we *hadn't* tried!

That night, a roomful of strangers whom I would never see again simply *heard* us. I tearfully told what life had been like for us recently. Dan shared his pain, too. Unlike anyone else, however, *they* heard us with ears molded by their own unique, but similar, pain. Afterward, for the first night in months, I actually experience some real sleep. We decided to continue to avail ourselves of this support when we returned home. We also were open to learning the Twelve Steps. We still had much to learn about the very first step- realizing that we were, and are, powerless over our own child!

Upon our return, we met a calm Burt. We told him he could either leave home and keep the check I had written, or stay at home and live by house rules. We didn't know when to quit! Living by house rules meant he would have to flush a quarter of a pound of "pot" down the toilet. We watched as he flushed three hundred and fifty dollars worth (dealer's cost) of marijuana into our septic tank, several bags at a time. (He later confessed that he seriously considered lifting the lid of the septic tank to fish some of it out!).

The year which followed is a blur. I recall attending Alanon and Narcotics Anonymous Family

Support meetings. I came to realize that I had led a very sheltered life. As bad as I felt, I still came to prefer our problem to that of anyone else. I also felt very moved by the honesty which I experienced. There was such beauty in seeing folks who were not trying to pretend to be something they were not. It was a refreshing contrast. I began also to see to what extent we *all* attempt to fool ourselves. What a high price we pay!

We were making progress in our own recovery; however, it was very slow. We actually made a loan to Burt so he could attend the local community college. We discovered later he would drive to the school parking lot and...sleep! We also attended family counseling sessions. Burt cooperated when he felt like it. We had arguments and one physical fight between Burt and Dan over going to counseling sessions. Finally, the family counselor suggested Burt might want to get some information from a substance abuse counselor. Burt met with this man who was a recovering addict, himself, several times; however, nothing seemed to make any difference in his behavior.

During this time, Burt was supposed to be having regular meetings with his probation officer. He would meet with her once, skip the next meeting, and postpone the one after that. He expected this would be acceptable. For many months, it was.

There came a day, however, when our family counselor, Burt's substance abuse counselor, his probation officer, and his parents all had an appointment to sit down together with him . Once again, Burt failed to appear. We held the meeting anyway. We each expressed our concerns. Burt was not following through on *any* of the commitments he had made.

After each of us had expressed our frustrations, Dan turned to Burt's probation officer. "I have to hold *you* responsible for some of this," he said. She seemed a bit shocked. "When Burt missed the very first appointment," Dan continued, 'you told him this was his first warning. You indicated that after a total of three warnings, you would have no choice but to file against him for probation violation. Yet, you have done nothing. All you are doing is teaching Burt that you don't mean what you say. Either don't threaten him or make good on your threats!" She admitted he was right. I doubt very much anyone had ever addressed this issue with her.

Another meeting was scheduled with the family counselor, the drug counselor, Burt , Dan, and myself. This time Burt *was* present. the counselors told Burt they were stopping treatment because he was not ready. When he *was* ready, he would know where to find them. The termination of counseling was another way of letting Burt go, of not trying to control him. It was *extremely* painful for us, his parents. Burt seemed neither relieved nor resentful about all of the comments on his behavior. He was simply oblivious. We were losing him.

From that day it became impossible to coexist within the same home. We were no longer able to deny the subtle indications that he was breaking every rule we had made in our mutual agreement. The indications were no longer subtle, but blatant, practically *begging* for consequences.

Reluctantly, we told Burt we were giving him one month to find another place to live. He agreed this would be best for all of us. In reality, he did absolutely nothing about it. Meanwhile, he assured us he was "working on it." On the appointed moving day, he announced to us that he had no place to go.

This was what we had dreaded. There was no turning back, now. We had two choices: continue to allow him to disrespect and abuse us or force him to leave home. We told him, as far as we were concerned, he could either go live with his friends (whom we knew were all using and selling drugs) or live in his car. We informed him he would have to leave the very next day. "Okay," he replied, always determined to give the appearance of being in control, "if that's the way it's going to be, *I'll leave right now!*"

When I hear stories of families who report that they "kicked their children out," my heart twists. I cannot know how it is for others, I only know that for us, it went against every parental instinct we have. We knew if we did not force him to leave, we were in almost certain danger of losing him to the final state of addiction which includes death, insanity or incarceration. We knew that if we *did* force him to leave, we ran the same risk. Paradoxically, we knew this was our only hope.

Only in living with the consequences of his behavior would Burt ever have a chance of recovering from addiction. We hoped and prayed the immediate consequences would not be too severe so he would have the opportunity for the self-awareness necessary to begin a journey into recovery.

At this point, as his loving parents, we knew we had done everything possible within our power. It was time for us to surrender. We were not giving up on our son, nor were we "kicking him out" like a piece of trash. We were simply acknowledging the reality that we *had* no control. We also realized *he* had no control. He would eventually have to choose whether or not he wished to create order from his own chaos. Painful as it was, giving him that choice was our gift to him.

***

CHAPTER NINE

When the time comes for something dreaded to happen, it usually does not take place in the way I have always feared it would. Reality is much less dramatic than fantasy. In the words of the poet, T. S. Eliot, "This is the way the world ends- not with a bang, but a whimper."

It was October. Just before dark, Burt came into the house highly agitated to find me stuffing his possessions into bags. "All right," he boomed, "I'll go But, first, I have to check on something. " I heard the car tires squeal as he roared out of the driveway. Fifteen minutes later, he phoned to announce that he was going to drive himself into a tree at eighty miles an hour. I heard my voice as though it were coming from another body, "Do whatever you have to do, Burt," I said.

I felt like two people- this disembodied voice which did not waver insulated by a thick resolve, and underneath, a quavering ball of fear.

Ten minutes later, Burt returned. He grabbed a few possessions and the three of us hugged. We told him we hoped he would remember what we had tried to teach him. We told him we loved him very much. He told us he loved us, too. Then he was gone.

For the next two months, I went through the motions of living. I ate. I worked. I went out with friends. I even laughed. I probably slept better because no one was pulling a car into the driveway with lights and noise in the middle of the night. Ignorance *was* bliss. What I didn't know had less power to hurt me. But now and then, the reality would come crashing through. I would stare at the photos of our children growing up. I grieved almost as though Burt had died.

Every few days, by chance, I might run into him on the street, walking or driving. He would give me a friendly wave. I would wave back, recognizing him, but wondering *who* was this, to whom was I waving?

One early morning around seven o'clock, Dan and I decided to go out for breakfast. As we were leaving the house, we encountered Burt. He was sitting forlornly in his car. We invited him to join us for breakfast. He politely declined, saying he felt too ill. "I'm scared," he said. "What are you afraid of" I asked him. "I did something last night," he answered. (It was remarkable, I thought, how calm I managed to remain). "What did you do, Burt?" "Well, does a razor blade and a mirror mean anything to you?" he riddled, clearly needing to talk with us, but extremely uncomfortable with the topic. *This*, I thought, is significant. "No, Burt, I'm sorry; it doesn't." "Mom and dad," he agonized, "I did cocaine last night, and I'm having a bad time right now." "Burt," I continued, as though he were explaining he had received a bad test score, "have you considered that you may have a problem with drugs?" "Well-I..." he replied, "I do know I'm considered prone to psychological addiction," (maybe all the counseling and the aborted stay in the drug rehab were not wasted after all, I thought). I remained as objective as possible. I weighed each word, "Burt, you know your father has diabetes. He has to take insulin and watch his diet. He can't "do" sweets. It's not his fault; it's just the way it is." "I know," he replied.

"I'm locked out of the apartment and the guys can't hear me knocking to get in. It's cold in the car. May I just sleep in the house for awhile?" I answered, "You can come in to make a phone call to your drug counselor and to get a warm jacket, but you may not stay and sleep."

Burt came into the house, made a phone call to his substance abuse counselor's answering service and left a message. I didn't believe he would follow it through, but, I did believe I saw a necessary process taking place. As he got a warm jacket out of the closet and prepared to leave, I said to him, "Burt, it is very painful for us to see you suffer; but, we are glad for this pain because you can learn from it. We love you and we know you need this pain." He left.

Years later, I was in the middle of writing my account of our experience. Burt was helping me with some of the details. As he read over the preceding account he said, "Mom, I didn't just *do* cocaine, I did a *lot* of cocaine!" I became aware of how insulated I am as a person who has had no experience with illegal drugs. "Educate me, Burt," I requested. He explained to me that "recreational users" of cocaine usually ingest about one half gram or fifty dollars worth. On that particular occasion, Burt had consumed as much as seven grams! He explained he had done two "eight balls" with three and one half grams in each one. This amounts to one quarter ounce of cocaine which in the late 1980's was valued at over five hundred dollars. He must have realized that his life was in imminent danger when he came over that morning. It is a miracle that he lived through the episode!

Burt also took this opportunity to depict the escalation of his drug use. He told me the very first time he did cocaine he did not like it. He was at college. It wound him up so much he couldn't sleep all night. Recalling Burt's earlier days, I knew one thing for certain: Burt did not need to be wound up! Two weeks after leaving home he tried cocaine again. Evidently, he liked it better this time. Burt described a pattern of exponential acceleration in his drug use. He would tell himself he would limit use to weekends. This lasted about two weeks. Then, he decided every half week would be better. Not long after that, every other day seemed a better plan. Soon, every day he was putting one eight ball of three and one half grams of cocaine into his body at a dealer's cost of two hundred dollars per day. This progression took all of two and one half months!

One other incident stands out in my mind. He phoned us from a motel room. He had been doing cocaine for two days and needed a ride because he didn't feel well enough to drive. We anguished over helping him. Dan feared he might have an accident and kill or injure someone. While this was a possibility, we had relapsed somewhat. The truth was, we were afraid *he'd* be killed or that he would be held responsible for someone else's demise. It was almost impossible to remove ourselves completely from being involved with Burt and his problem as long as we had any awareness that he was in some kind of trouble.

***

CHAPTER TEN

Our awareness was about to change. When we left for Thanksgiving in November and drove on to Florida, we were unknowingly creating a situation where we were not available. It was during the month's time period when Burt was steadily using cocaine. Burt finally missed one-too-many probation appointments. He doesn't remember very much else that entire month.

November 30th, 1988, Dan's birthday. As we toured the retired aircraft carrier, The Lexington, in Pensacola with our son, daughter and her family, Burt was being arrested and taken to jail. It is the anniversary of his sobriety.

For some reason, he stopped using even though drugs were available from within the jail. Not that he thought he had a problem! After our initial tearful reunion in a visiting cell across a wooden table among a roomful other jail inmates, we were astounded to hear his reasoning. His focus was entirely on *his* rights being violated! He detailed to us his research in the jail library. He informed us of the other inmates' expert opinions on how the authorities had done him dirt. Rather than attempting to dissuade him, we simply listened. We seemed to realize there was something very desperate and disturbed, almost delusional, in his logic. We intuited it would not only be useless to argue with him; it would somehow encourage his defensiveness.

Visiting hours at the jail were twice a week. In order to ensure you would be admitted into the visitors' room, you had to arrive at least a half hour early. You had to wait in line in the "holding tank"- a sort of vestibule to the main door. It was winter and line overflowed outside, so if you were first, you were able to be warm! After realizing this was going to be a necessary ritual, we began to look for anything which would make the experience interesting.

I will never forget the folks I met, some quite regularly, the tiny children, the unusual conversations. Sometimes, I actually miss this ritual which contained within it a microcosm of human living- all that is bad and good about life. At the appointed time, the door buzzed and we "made it through the count" to the waiting room. There was a limit on the number of people who could be in the tiny visitors' room at one time. Once in the waiting room, it was necessary to sign in and meet with the guard's approval. There we were, this humble cadre of humanity, lined up to be electronically scanned and sometimes physically frisked so that we might have the privilege of encountering and embracing our loved ones who had, to one degree or another, run afoul of the law. Burt's "afoulness" in violating probation terms by not keeping appointments was probably the *mildest* infraction; murder was the most severe.

We hardly ever missed a visiting day. We returned early from out-of-town trips so we could get to the jail for our visit. We wrote almost every day, did the wash, and took care of any possible requests. Judging from the odor of Burt's dirty laundry, the smell of the place, alone would have been punishment enough for me!

We had no expectations. We had no idea what would happen when Burt finished four months of his sentence. After we accepted the fact that Burt was in jail, we were able to relax because he seemed to be safer *there* than he had been living on his own!

We began to concentrate on caring for ourselves. Family members were very supportive. The sustaining power of friends was immensely appreciated. We continued to attend Alanon and NA Family Group meetings. We were touched by many kind gestures of folks we knew only slightly.

Then to our amazement, one February day after Burt had been in jail for two and one half months, he suddenly remarked, "You know? I've been thinking.

Maybe it *is* me. Maybe I'm not thinking right. Maybe I *do* need help. Do you think the help you offered to me before might still be available?" It was as though he had walked around the huge wall of denial and could stand for a moment where we were standing.

We knew better than to be elated or ecstatic. But, we felt very, very hopeful. We decided to wait and see if his insight lasted. He began to attend meetings of Alcoholics and Narcotics Anonymous in the jail.

We realized the AA and NA meetings were one way to escape boredom. At this point, we didn't care if he was totally serious about seeing his reality or not, as long as he went to the meetings. When Burt's attitude proved to be consistent, we asked him if he would like to begin preparations for treatment placement. He was relieved. Perhaps this was the "readiness" he needed to have. We arranged for his substance abuse counselor to meet with him in jail.

When Burt completed his jail term, we were permitted to drive him directly upon his release from jail to the same rehab he had been to before. We stopped once- for a haircut, lunch and new clothing. It was the day after Easter Sunday, March 29th, 1989. He changed into his new clothing. We stopped along the way to take a photograph of him standing, very symbolically, in front of a cemetery-Burt's resurrection!

***

CHAPTER ELEVEN

After all we had experienced, we still did not fully understand this disease of addiction. WE thought now that he was no longer in denial and knew he had a problem with substances, all he needed was one month in a rehab. And so did he!

We were puzzled that he seemed to be sleepy most of the time in treatment. We did not see him during the week, but we visited with him each Saturday and also participated in family treatment exercise. His counselors simply would not accept his sleepiness. Burt said the sleepiness just kept coming over him so he couldn't concentrate or get to compulsory meetings on time. Nevertheless, at the end of the "Family Four Day Intensive Program" run by this particular treatment center, Burt was finally able to be fully honest for the first time about the extent of his drug habit and the outrageous behaviors which accompanied it.

"Mom and dad," he began, "when you're on cocaine, you think you are all powerful. You think you can do *anything*! " He proceeded to tell us hair-raising tales of being a drug-runner in and out of New York City and of Jamaican gangs with automatic weapons. He told us that he, himself, had been carrying a gun. "You feel powerful, like one of the characters in a television crime show!"

I could suddenly see clearly the connection between what kids today are puffing and snorting with their lips and nose and what they are devouring with their eyes from the violent dare-devil antics seen on TV. Get the idea from TV and act it out with a little help from your drug of choice!

Burt told us of having been stopped by a police officer for speeding one day after his driver's license had expired. He was transporting two kilos of cocaine. *Two kilos*! This is an *enormous* amount. The dealer's cost for this amount of cocaine was thirty four thousand

Necessary Steps : A Family's Journey

dollars. Sold in eight balls, it would bring in at least one hundred and ninety seven thousand dollars! One cannot get much closer to "living on the edge." The cocaine was not discovered. Amazing Grace! We were incredulous!! Thank God we received this information when we were capable of handling it psychologically and emotionally.

After completing the four week treatment program, Burt was eager to return home. He said he wanted to attend post treatment, outpatient clinics run by the treatment center and connect with local AA and NA groups. This sounded very reasonable. However, the treatment center's recommendation was for more extensive, in-patient treatment. The probation officer insisted Burt abide by the treatment center's recommendations. Counselors from the center took Burt on a tour of a treatment home where rigorous treatment with many strict rules lasted for eighteen months to two years.

Burt rebelled. He'd had enough! We later learned addictive personalities often do not know what they need, only what they want. Perhaps this could be said of most people to some degree. With addicts, it is certainly true to a far *greater* degree.

Once again we were in the narrow, vice-like grip of another necessary process. With the help of Burt's counselor, we came up with an alternative- a therapeutic community made up of teens and young people with parents heavily engaged in treatment. The parents also helped to run the program. There was no set time limit of treatment duration. Families stayed until it was decided by the staff that they were ready to graduate.

This therapeutic community, known also as a "TC," was a drive of four hours from our home. Burt would have to stay in the geographical area of the TC. In the first phase of treatment, all the kids stayed in a "host" home with parents who also had a child in the program. After the initial phase, children returned home to live and to work on family interactions. However because of the distance in our case, Burt would have to continue to board with a host home for most of the program. We would be expected to come for training and treatment in a parent group- twice a week in the initial treatment stages and once a week as progress was made. Eventually, we would get to know other parents and possibly also stay in a host home for the weekend.

We liked the idea of a family component, but we were intimidated by the distance! However, we would have done anything in our power to prevent Burt from having to go to state prison. Moreover, after all we had been through, and despite the positive path Burt appeared to be on, the probation officer was adamant that Burt be required to go on for extended treatment as recommended. Otherwise, he would once again be considered "in violation." *This* time, he would probably be sentenced to a year in the state penitentiary for failing to cooperate with treatment recommendations!

Once again, the situation was completely out of our hands. Ironically, frustrating as this was for us, this is *exactly* where it needed to be.

On the phone that last night, calling us from the treatment center, Burt announced to us that he was not going to *either* long-term program.

It was as though I were in a recurring nightmare- the kind where someone is chasing you and you cannot run or scream for help. I felt like a large beetle on its back with legs flailing! Dan rose to the challenge, however. I heard him say in an even-toned voice with almost no emotion, "Burt, you must choose. Either you are going to the long-term program recommended by the treatment center or the flexible time therapeutic community which was found with the help of your counselor. The other thing you can do is to go to state prison. If you choose the last option, we will not be visiting you this time."

There was an excruciatingly long silence.

Then, through the sound of my heart thumping in my chest, I heard, "Okay, I'll go to that program you found in Massachusetts."

***

CHAPTER TWELVE

On the day Burt was discharged, exactly one month from the day he entered the treatment center, we drove him directly to the program we had found.

Later, we heard stories from parents who had tricked their kids into treatment in this program. They felt they had to do whatever it took to get their kids there, because they were literally killing themselves with chemicals and dangerous behaviors. By contrast, since Burt was already partially into recovery, he came with us willingly once he accepted the decision. True, he had not wanted to go, but we were confident that our firm stand, once again, was the right one.

Burt was interviewed by a pleasant young woman who administered the MAST (Michigan Alcohol Screening Test). He agreed with her about the results. Before beginning recovery he had been at the final state which includes death, insanity or incarceration. He turned over his jewelry and his belt to us, gave us hugs and was led away by two young men who were holding on to his belt loops. They would be with him, watching his every move for many days to come.

Most of the parents who brought their children to this program had to contend with verbal and physical abuse as they prepared to leave their children.

It was necessary to physically restrain many of these youngsters to prevent them from injuring themselves or others or doing damage to the building, a converted warehouse which housed the daytime sessions of the program. In each case, they were carefully restrained by other young people who were further along in the program. I was very impressed with the way in which the restraining was done. I began to see it served a purpose beyond holding a young person down. It served to calm and even comfort, as well as capture. It was the restraining parents of young children do when they refuse to allow their toddlers to run into a busy street!

Just as illegal drugs have become a big business, so have rehabilitation centers! A month at a private "in-house" rehabilitation facility can cost over twelve thousand dollars. This is covered by health insurance. We were extremely fortunate to have health insurance. It took care of almost all of the costs of Burt's first treatment facility- *both times*!

The second treatment facility, the TC, made Burt's first rehab look like a posh country club. Whereas the in-house facility was housed in beautiful buildings in an idyllic rural setting, the TC held day meetings in a former warehouse. At the rehab, Burt had a schedule of group meetings and lectures. However, there was also a gym and an Olympic size swimming pool. He was permitted to smoke ("we can't tackle all addictions at once!" was the logic). All he really had to do was learn information from movies and lectures and share information in group sessions over coffee in comfortable lounges. The TC, by contrast, was more like "boot camp!" In the first setting, Burt learned the Twelve Steps of Alcoholics Anonymous; in the second setting, he *lived* them.

In the late 1970's a group of concerned parents and professionals came together with the idea of developing a non-profit, comprehensive treatment program for addicted adolescents and their families. They made no distinction between alcohol, heroin, marijuana or cocaine. They regarded addiction, itself, to be a treatable condition. The drug-using and other damaging behaviors engaged in by young addicts were viewed as symptoms of this fundamental addiction.

They developed a structured, self-help program in which the kids would help the kids and the parents would help the parents. Families would be helpers and role models for each other as they progressed through a carefully designed program of earned stages. While professionals were used, they were peripheral. Eventually, these centers spread geographically. At one time there were eight of them scattered through the United States.

It is not possible to establish branches of this TC in many states due to legal restrictions. For instance, the age at which a child is legally emancipated must be as low as possible. If a child is considered emancipated legally at the age of sixteen, a parent may not place the child in treatment against his or her will after this age. There are also legal requirements which make placing children in homes other than their parents difficult. This was done at our TC by screening each family to become formal foster parents within the state social welfare system.

The ideal situation would be that everyone who started the program would stick it out; however, that was not the case. Therefore, families would drop out of the program suddenly and it would be necessary to place their wards in another home. This could happen at any time and most state foster care systems are not set up for such constantly changing conditions.

This is so different from most people's concept of a drug treatment facility where the family simply drops off their child and picks him or her up four to seven weeks later. In those facilities, usually on the weekend, there may be family treatment consisting of a few movies and a couple of discussion groups. There may also be an optional few days of more intensive group treatment which merely scratches the surface of how the family maintains an environment which creates the conditions for addiction.

The standard rehabilitation facility requires very little from the adolescent or the family. While young people are told it is their responsibility to maintain their sobriety, the behavioral message from the facility is that this *is* "the cure." There is after treatment available at the standard facility and perhaps by the third or fourth time through such a treatment facility, one realizes that one had better continue into after treatment! Before our experience with Burt, I actually believed one could spend four to seven weeks in such a facility and find this sufficient for overcoming one's addiction! When Burt went through his four weeks, he encountered people who had been through the program up to *seven times*!

Why is it rehab centers generally set two to four weeks for the duration of their recovery program (seven for adolescents)? For one reason. It is the amount of time covered by insurance companies.

Many families entered the TC expecting to be involved in the same way as in these four week or seven week treatment centers. Even the folks who lived with in a half hour of the program felt overwhelmed by this program's demands. The program consumed the entire lives of the kids and their parents. For some parents, this was simply too much! Due to ignorance of what they were sacrificing or though misplaced

Necessary Steps : A Family's Journey

values or conscious choice, many of them removed themselves in the first weeks or months. Too much was required. The parents' unwillingness to undergo change paralleled their kids' refusal to give up using substances. Moreover, many of the parents, themselves, were in denial about their *own* chemical dependency and other compulsive behaviors! Eventually, it became clear to informed observers that the entire family was trapped in a rigid, addictive pattern which fostered and fertilized their youngster's drug problem.

The TC relied heavily upon the positive use of peer pressure to change behaviors in both the kids and the parents. Based on the idea that it was peer pressure which first got a kid involved with drugs, supervised peer pressure was used to help the youngsters get off and stay off drugs. One of the toughest parts of treatment for parents was the focusing of the adult peer pressure on their individual and couple behaviors. If a family remained in the program after the first few weeks, they would unquestioningly be subjected to this adult peer pressure. By that time, bonds had been established with many or the parents which was the only thing which made this pressure palatable.

In order to accept recommendations which came from the parent group, an individual had to be willing to invest the group with an almost parental authority. One had to be able to trust in the group as their "higher power" with a consensual ability to perceive an individual's real needs accurately. Many of these folks came from homes in which their parents could not be trusted in this way. It took many months of building trust before most people felt comfortable trusting the parent group as their authority. In the same way, it took time for the kids to learn to trust their young people's group.

Over a period of months, Burt had to work his way through group processes to earn any privilege he received. Upon entry, he was required to surrender all his possessions. He could wear only T shirts without slogans. Jewelry was not permitted, and he was strongly encouraged to have a short hair cut. He could not smoke. Initially, he could not talk to girls. He had to give up his privacy. Another young man in the program, but a bit further along, was given the responsibility of "shadowing" Burt every moment from the time he got up in the morning until he went to bed at night, even accompanying him to the bathroom! In the beginning he had to request permission at meals to pick up an eating utensil! He had to learn how to survive in a completely new culture. Once before in his life, he and his family had been in such a situation.

Burt was only three when we went for our two year company assignment in the Netherlands. Each day we awoke in a strange country. When we were in public, we were surrounded with the sounds of a strange language. Initially, we struggled with an unfamiliar currency and a new system of weights and measures. Gradually, we adjusted to the differences and began to learn the language enough to function comfortably.

Our children were already very close, but they became even closer as they shared this extraordinary experience. The older two went to an International School in Amsterdam. There, they made friends with children from many different countries. In their home neighborhood, they played with Dutch children and learned to speak the Dutch language fairly well. I remember Leanne, age thirteen, in her position as bus monitor, giving directions to the location of the school in Dutch to a new driver while keeping a watchful eye out for misbehaving students. It occurs to me this is not entirely unrelated to her present role as parish minister and pastor of a city congregation!

It was a fascinating, mind-stretching experience. We had to change our behavior to accommodate to this different culture. This is exactly what it was like for all of us to be part of the TC.

For many families, this TC was their last hope. They had already been through traditional rehabilitation centers, alcohol treatment centers and psychiatric facilities. After a few months, it became clear to us why one month in a traditional rehab is only a beginning. In almost every case, including our own, the young people who were thought to be "offenders" by their families and by society were only the iceberg's tip. The entire family system needed to be restructured to some degree in every case. This process would require months, perhaps *years* of all-out effort by every family member.

The habits of past generations- the unspoken rules of "culture" of our ancestors dictate the behavior of every family system. This TC sought nothing less than to bring about the healthy redesign of whole family systems. The kids had a group, the parents had a group, and the siblings had a group. Each individual learned the basic philosophy of the culture through rules and slogans which were based on the Twelve Steps. Each group then used this basic learning as the foundation from which the group could create more rules as needed for relating to each other and to the other groups. Special terms were used to describe practices used with the TC. Again, we were learning a new language. And, just as in the Netherlands, we found ourselves bonding very quickly with other Americans because we were all strangers in a strange country, in the TC we found that same magnetism. Families whose children have been caught up in the drug culture are desperate to connect and relate to other such families. We were akin to being "fox hole buddies" in the battle for our children's lives!

Our friends at home thought we had joined a cult. Our behavior, our speech, even the songs we sang during the large meetings which began every parent-child session reflected our new alliance. Our emotions were totally on the surface. We no longer "fit" into "polite society." We became *real*. We knew what mattered!

Some of the tactics which this TC employed have been attacked by groups in American society who feel strongly about an individual's civil rights. It is true such behaviors as the "boot camp" maneuvers *are* reprehensible when the intention is to oppress people. However, when the intention is to motivate people to give up old, destructive behaviors and replace them with new, healthy ones, they are of inestimable value.

There were two settings for learning healthy behaviors: the warehouse for day treatment and the host homes where the young people stayed overnight. Each family had staying with them one young person who had been around long enough to take responsibility for the newer young people. This was a huge task for that young person, not *unlike* parenting! The kids were never locked in; they were alarmed in- that is, if anyone bolted through the door or windows, a buzzer would automatically warn the household that this was happening. (Area hardware stores did a brisk business...). This newly responsible young person known as the "Oldcomer," was challenged to go after the "bolter" and bring the person back!

At one point in treatment at the TC Burt had earned the position of "Oldcomer." He was looking out for a "Newcomer," a young man about four years younger than Burt. He invested so much of himself into trying to help Chuck see the errors of his addictive thinking. Many times, Chuck tested the limits of everyone in the program, both counselors and clients. He would stage a rumpus, start a fight, or run away. This behavior escalated to the point where even restraining failed. Some of Chuck's antics let to broken bones.

While Burt did not experience lasting physical injury due to Chuck's wild thrashing out, he was terribly hurt emotionally. He had earned the right to spend free time with us and he used to confide in us how frustrating and painful it was to attempt to control this wild young man. Many times, he broke down and wept. "What a beautiful program this is," I said to my husband, "for in dealing with Chuck, Burt is living out the hell he put *us* through." By the time he was finished with this TC, he had experienced every angle of an addictive system from the chemical dependency side to the codependent facets. This treatment system simply redid life!

Each day there were chores for the kids to do at home. There might be three to five kids in one host home so, needless to say, that alone acted to change family dynamics.

Boys and girls in the program did not mix in the host homes. There were boy host homes and girl host homes. Of course, if a boy in the program had a sister or sisters, they would be in the home, also and vice-versa.

Somehow, what kids will not do for their parents, they will do for other parents, host parents. The ingenious part was their care-taking mentor, their Oldcomer. The kids learned the healthy new behaviors from their peers- those who are most influential in their lives at this stage of development. Each evening before going to bed, each young person had to write a kind of report on himself based on how he or she had applied the Twelve Steps to living that Day. It was called a "Moral Inventory. All of the parents had to do the same in the initial training stages. They were encouraged to continue this through the course of the program.

Since we lived too far away to have any young people living in our home, we served as surrogate parents on weekends. The regular host parents needed a break and we needed the experience of serving as host parents.

What a unique experience! Imagine yourself suddenly materializing in a strange kitchen. It is your responsibility to create a meal out of whatever is in the refrigerator. You know the rules: no knives or other sharp objects left out in the open, no vanilla flavoring (it is thirty nine percent alcohol), no doors or windows left unalarmed. This week, the staff has informed the parents that no cookies, cakes or carbonated beverages are permitted; the kids are too wound up. The kids will test you. They will insist the rules were changed and now it's okay. You must be prepared to say a firm, "No." You may or may not know the kids. Someone new may be arriving. Mentally and emotionally, you prepare yourself. You are the mom!

The door opens and five young men fairly fall into the room weighted down with knapsacks and notebooks. Two of them are physically hooked together, fingers through belt loops. "Hi, mom, how're ya doin'?" yells a tired, but cheerful young man. He herds his charges in front of him. "Okay, door's closed, alarm's on," calls my husband, Dan, the dad. "Whew," the young man breathes. He relaxes his hold on the "Newcomer." It is the Newcomer's first day in the program. His eyes are wide with fright. He looks as though he has just landed on another planet!

Once inside an alarmed house, most youngsters behave. They may have "acted out" like mad animals at the program all day; however, in the company of their peers and two strange adults, they conform in the home. Why is this? Could it be young people mainly need to feel secure, accepted and guided?

Dinner is pizza. Simple to make and simple to clean up. The boys take care of the mess under the direction of their "Oldcomer."

After chores are done, the boys write their "moral inventories" according to the Twelve Steps. You help them. They seem so vulnerable and so in need of nurturing it is impossible *not* to love them. There is not much for you to do other than simply be there. When they are finished, the Oldcomer takes over and shepherds everyone back to their sleeping room.

That night, you sleep in a strange bed in a strange bedroom. You feel like you, *too*, are on another planet! The next morning, while you put a simple breakfast on the table, the Oldcomer makes sure the boys are ready to be driven to their day treatment. No mother of normal teens ever had it so easy. This is the home portion of the program, running smoothly.

Our weekend surrogate parenting experiences *did* go smoothly. We did not encounter some of the situations with which the regular parents had to struggle. No one ran away or attempted suicide on our "watch." Nevertheless, it was comforting to know help was as close as our phone should we need it.

During our tenure, we were called upon by parents to assist. We often drove one or two hours to be with other families who were in crisis. If a child took off, the dads and moms would search for the runaway. Most of the time, they were found and returned to the program. Sometimes they were not found. Sometimes families simply dropped out. If they returned, they were placed on a "set back" for several days or weeks. They had to start at the beginning and slowly re-earn all their privileges. Some of them had to learn the same lesson over and over and over. The program was a microcosm of life!

Each week, we would attend a large, combined meeting of the kids and their parents . We would have a chance to see how the kids were doing and how the parents were relating to the kids. Various young people in different stages of recovery would tell their stories. The parents would share their experiences. Finally, the new kids would explain how they came to be there. Some were as young as twelve. They would tell of the drinking they had done and the other drugs they had used. They would tell about some of the problems their behavior created. Each story seemed more shocking and incredible than the last one.

Saying these things to a roomful of people made it impossible to deny what people had been doing to themselves. Hearing what was said by others made them aware they were not the only ones in a similar predicament.

When defenses between human beings are removed, we can see in reality we are not separate. It is a paradox: we are unique individuals; yet, at the same time, *we are all one*. I can recognize *my* pain in you and *your* pain in me. We can be honest with one another. The truth really does set us free! It is enough, then, to be ourselves- neither less nor more than who we truly are.

After the large, combined meeting we would have our parent group meeting while the kids had one of their own on the other side of a divided room.

Simultaneously, the sibling group would meet in another section of the building.

Parents who were further along in the program took turns monitoring the sibling group. On the few occasions where I assisted, I was very impressed with the seriousness with which these mostly pre-teens conducted their meetings. There was a natural order of leadership among them according to the amount of experience and length of time in the program. I could not help but think of the benefits these kids were deriving from having to deal with their family crises.

These young people were dealing with crucial issues, moral issues. Children used to learn these things at home from their parents and grandparents, aunts and uncles. Religious teachings affirmed them. At the present time, with too few exceptions, the families of our nation are floundering in amorality in my opinion. Parents and children, alike, are doing whatever seems right or feels good in the moment without regard to long-term consequences. All of the traditional values have undergone a remarkable shift and the line between right and wrong has become blurred. People in positions of authority have engaged in misleading behavior and outright deceit!

As I write these words, a portion of Handel's "Messiah" runs through my head: "All we like sheep have gone astray, every one to his own way." I wonder what poetry and music runs through the minds of today's children? What do they find of value? What makes life worthwhile for them? What will become their passion in life? I recall a message I recently read from a roadside billboard: "If you don't know what you stand for, you'll fall for anything." There is a great deal of "anything" out there in the world ready to rush in and fill up the vacuum, the empty spot where our Higher Power should be! With all of the scientific and technical advancements of the past century, will our descendants still look back upon this era in time as a second "Dark Ages?"

I love freedom. I hate to be told what to do or how to think! I would rather sort through ideas and choose my own opinions. But, I have become aware that within my lifetime in the name of freedom people are enslaving themselves! *Without self-discipline there can be no freedom.* It seems most of our nation's homes have minimal ability to discipline children. As a result, a great many of our nation's schools reflect this inability to discipline. The schools cannot do it if the parents cannot do it. How then will young people develop the ability to discipline and regulate themselves?

Perhaps there has been and always will be a segment of the younger generation which seems like an agricultural crop grown wild! It may be an illusion which has come upon me in mid-life; but, this segment seems to be increasing in numbers and in influence. Why is this happening?

In my adult lifetime, I have experienced the erosion of respect within every social institution beginning with the family and followed by churches, schools, business, government, and the legal system.

Perhaps there is an arrogance in the presumption human beings can improve on nature. As a species, we have always attempted to superimpose our own brand of order upon the world. We seem doomed to struggle in order to prevent chaos. In so doing we *create* our own chaos! Our downfall as a species comes, however, from our tendency to develop one set of orderly beliefs and then behave in direct opposition to our stated principles. This hypocrisy has been occurring in recorded history since the days of Moses! It seems to be an indispensable part of human nature.

Paul, the Christian apostle, wrote "That which I should do, I do not, and that which I should not do, I do." We go against our better instincts and intentions. In Christian theology this is the concept of "original sin." It is certainly evident in the world regardless of one's religious beliefs.

It occurs to me that chaos, itself, is neither good nor bad. It just is. There are even theories that chaos, if examined minutely, contains order within itself. What is destructive, however, is hypocrisy: stating a belief and acting out its opposite! Apply this to one social institution: education.

Every year since my adolescence the SAT scores of American students have fallen. Every year, the touted solution to this problem has been increased spending. No matter how much money is spent, the scores continue on a downward trend while parents and educators wring their hands in collective consternation. Today, this is seen by many educators, businessmen and politicians as in intractable problem.

Does anyone really believe today's generation of young Americans is less intelligent, less creative than its predecessors? No. The problem is not one of innate ability. Are they perhaps less motivated? Are they too complacent? Are they overwhelmed with all of the economic, political and social changes? Perhaps these are factors. However, I suggest the bottom line has to do with respect. Respect can't be bought. It is not for sale. It must be expected. It must be taught. It must be earned. If children have little respect for their parents and teachers, they will have little respect for themselves. Not surprisingly, self-respect is tied directly to self-discipline.

When I substituted in public high schools, I heard the principal over the loudspeaker request the kids to rise for the pledge of allegiance to the flag. I witnessed children grudgingly stand up, slumping, fidgeting, and talking through the whole ceremony. This is a small thing, but it is *not* trivial. If this is done with disrespect, it would be better if it were not done at all. To do this small thing without respect teaches incongruity and disintegrity in one small act which is repeated daily in our public schools. Such small acts generalize to larger ways of thinking and behaving.

We are not aware of the significance these rituals and ceremonies have for our lives. The danger is not so much in giving them up; it is in doing them without respect. This is only one way in which we imply to our children that respect for rituals, rules, and what used to be known as "good taste" is *optional* in our society. I believe contemporary society has lost its rituals or in many cases rendered them meaningless. We thought they were optional. They are *not!*

It was comforting to me to witness in the sibling group something like a positive version of "Lord of the Flies." I observed children who were doing for themselves what their parents and other influential adults had become unable to do for them- develop meaningful rules and rituals. In this way they would create self-discipline and ultimately self-respect. This was inspiring! I found myself wishing there were a way

Necessary Steps : A Family's Journey

for such groups to expand and flourish in schools and churches throughout the country and throughout the world.

Approval and disapproval of parents in the parent group conditioned weaker parents to set and abide by rules. They used these rules with the kids who lived with them, both their own and the other young people in the program. Infractions on both sides were dealt with in the respective groups. An acceptable format and process for communicating and receiving feedback concerning these infractions was learned in the initial training we received. In this way the ability to create discipline was slowly restored to parents. A positive way to deal with infractions was also learned. Our program trainers were parents who had graduated from the program.

This TC was far more economical as well as far more effective than the month long facility. The cost for one year in the TC was about the same as for one *month* in the rehab. Part of the cost of treatment was offset by fund-raising projects which the parent group sponsored and implemented. Not only did this raise needed money for the program; people also learned how to work together toward a common goal. The by-products of this included increased self-esteem, both individual and community, and camaraderie. Many people learned how to openly share themselves and their talents, some newly discovered, for the first time in their lives! I became aware that there are many people who, because they do not have blatant addiction problems, never have the opportunity to do this. What an unexpected blessing.

In our case we also paid a boarding fee in addition to the fee for the program. This was arranged between us and the host parents on a totally voluntary basis. The program was not covered by any insurance, mainly because of its unconventional method of housing the kids. Insurance companies pay only for treatment in an institutional setting. Since only the day treatment occurred in this setting and the children slept in private homes during the night, this program did not qualify despite the fact it has been proven to be far more economical and definitely more effective than a conventional fourteen to twenty eight day adult treatment program or a forty nine day adolescent treatment program.

In life it is a truism, the most expensive thing is not always the best! One thinks of the large amounts of money being paid out by insurance companies for a conventional drug treatment program. As stated previously, this is the *other* side of the drug business. We had to pay "up front" in the TC. This ensured families would not leave immediately when they became aware of how demanding this program would be. We took out a loan. We were still paying it off three years later. It was worth every penny!

***

CHAPTER THIRTEEN

The TC, alone, could be the subject of many books from several different perspectives. It could be studied sociologically and linguistically as well as from an addictions treatment point of view. As a family systems therapist, I received an invaluable education.

The difference between knowing the steps and living the steps became evident after Burt had been at the TC for about four months. He then told us when he was about to leave the first rehab it was in the back of his mind to go back to "just selling" drugs until he had "just enough" to set himself up in a nice apartment. Then, of course, he planned to quit having anything to do with illegal drugs. He was now able to pin-point his wrong, addictive thinking. We were tuning in to what a long, drawn-out process recovery is, especially in the first stages.

We received much we were not expecting through our involvement with the TC. In the beginning stage, Burt had to earn the right to spend just five minutes twice a week with us in a formally structured meeting. He did this by being cooperative in group meetings during the day treatment, participating in discussions in a positive manner. We had to limit our conversation to the events of the past and speak only of our individual feelings about them. Discussion of the present was prohibited. Mentors from both the kids' and the parents' groups were present to monitor the five minute conversation. Burt was not allowed any mail or phone calls.

His support system was thus taken away and he had to earn it back! As a result, *we* became incredibly precious to him. Naturally, *he* had been this precious to us since his birth. Now we had the basis for true appreciation of each other! We eagerly anticipated the day when he would earn the privilege of the rite of "home coming." Since we resided four hours from the area, he would not actually return home to live, but we would all be able to be together in a host home on the weekends. It was as though he were about to be born *again*. We were expectant parents!

None of the parents know when their child has earned this right to return home. During the large, combined group meeting, the child, who has learned this only a short time earlier, runs across a huge room into his parents outstretched arms. Perhaps I can best describe the immense power of this moment by witnessing that I am once again weeping tears of joy in reliving this as I write.

After this event in our lives, we were able to explore family dynamics on weekends. Sometimes this was done in regular family meetings (family "raps") involving whoever was in the house at the time, both the kids and the parents.

These meetings affirmed for us that everyone's family dynamics are basically the same. Each family has to learn to cope with the issues of each of its individual members. We adults bring to our present family all the "business" of our original families. Most of us bring along unmet dependency needs and feelings of low self esteem. This is not because we have had bad parenting, although most people *do* come from families with some degree of dysfunction. Our parents do the best job they know how in raising us. They can only "give as good as they got." The next generation either hands this on, or stops and takes a look at what works and what doesn't work. There is usually room for improvement. Probably every family could benefit from this evaluation, but in the case of a family with an addict, *it can make the difference between life and death!*

Living for many years as children in families where alcohol or other substance abuse or compulsive and addictive behaviors are the normal pattern, creates lasting scars. Even living with someone who is suffering from a chronic physical, mental, or emotional disorder can create unhealthy patterns of behavior in and among family members. Most of the time individuals are not even aware of these effects and, therefore, may deny having them.

Most people can come to an understanding of extremes in any situation. Typically, they also believe they share the same idea of what is normal. This assumption, however, may be far from the truth, depending upon each frame of reference. We use the word "normal" as though some kind of objective, universal, mathematical measure called "normalcy" exists. It comes as a complete surprise to many, and never to some, that *there is no normal.* There is only *your* normal and *my* normal. They may be worlds apart! Certainly, in any one, specific, measurable situation there will always be an average, but there *is* no generic normal!

People gravitate to what they know. The unfamiliar creates anxiety in human beings. Even the *worst* situations will be reproduced because, in a basic way, they are *known,* and therefore, safe. The patterns of response built around these situations are comfortable and familiar. In order for each of us to remain sane, reality *must* make sense. Strangely, what may appear to be extremely self-destructive or even bizarre behavior will make complete sense if we can only understand all of the factors. The "whole" really *is* the "sum of its parts."

However, some of the behaviors which people engage in to maintain familiar patterns create other problems. In this way, disease or "dis-ease" of one kind or another- either that of addiction or of codependency- perpetuates itself generation after generation.

Thus, it came as no surprise that there were areas in our own family which needed addressing. In our prior counseling, both as individuals and as a couple, I believe we had made some progress; however, I always felt there was much more to be resolved.

Imagine a fish tank, an aquarium. All the "mud" had sunk to the bottom of our family "fish tank." I could see while the water around us was clear, there was a lot of silt settled on the bottom. (This was preferable to constantly choking on mud). In order to deal with the mud, however, everyone had to *see* it! Something or someone had to *disturb* it. That someone was Burt. He kicked up the silt at the bottom of our family "fish tank!"

One Sunday, in a family "rap" meeting, Burt openly shared how he had turned to substances to experiment. He found they helped him feel more comfortable and relaxed in dealing with the inevitable anxieties of living life. He could avoid unpleasant feelings and feel "on top" of everything. When using drugs, he felt himself to be "in control" and, therefore, safe and secure. He described many aspects of his personality which he had come to know: his impatience with others, his perfectionism, his desire for exciting, even risky, activity which brought him a good, "high" feeling.

Later, when only the three of us were together, Dan told Burt he could identify with him. He acknowledged they were really very much alike. "*You* turned to drugs, Burt, and *I* turned to my work. Other than that, we're cut from the same mold!"

I never thought I would hear those words from my husband. I knew there had always been this tendency for Dan to "escape into work." It seemed to validate him and create a feeling of security for him. In our society it is the respectable addiction, difficult to challenge or confront. It is rewarded and encouraged. However, when taken to extremes or relied upon solely to provide us with false feelings of self-worth and security, it can become compulsive. It can kill- emotionally, spiritually, and even physically.

An invisible gap between father and son began to close that day.

Just as Dan was learning more about *him*self, *I* was learning also. Have you ever tried to see the back of your head without using a mirror or other reflecting surface? Obviously, this is impossible. What is not so obvious is that it is equally as difficult to see the way we really are as individuals. In order to do this, we need people to be truthful with us as to how we affect them. Counselors refer to this as "feedback."

We believe we can see ourselves objectively. After all, we certainly can see how other people harm themselves and alienate others! I prided myself on my ability to see this. I was, and still am, frequently correct. Consequently, it was very difficult for me not to tell my husband and my children what I saw. Naturally, I wanted to be helpful, and I wanted our lives together to work.

I saw myself as a loving, helpful person. But, what I could *not* see was how, particularly in a crisis, my desperate attempts to help sometimes got in the way. I was at these moments suffering from "controlitis." I came across at times like a "know-it-all." Frequently, the end result was that my unappreciative "helpees" greatly resented this "helping." Instead of me tending to my own needs and letting others do the same, we would all get into a cycle of manipulation and countermanipulation which left everyone totally frustrated.

The toughest part of this was I had to learn if another individual chooses *not* to attend to what I perceive as their need, it is *their* business, not mine. I had to relearn my role as wife and mother. I had to learn to live the Serenity Prayer: "God, grant me the serenity to accept the things I cannot change, the courage to change the things I can, and the wisdom to know the difference."

By openly sharing my experiences and feelings in groups at the TC, in counseling, in Codependency and Alanon groups and with an honest friend, I was finally able to glimpse "the back of my head." From time to time, I slip back into my old, control disease, but I am becoming much better at spotting it early and naming it for what it is. If you can name it, you can tame it!

***

CHAPTER FOURTEEN

The parent training portion of the TC included training in expressing emotions. In small groups of seven or eight people, parents were taught a "recipe" which I had learned in my counselor training courses in graduate school. I used it with my clients. It is deceptively simple. One wonders why anyone would *need* to learn it. That is, until you hear folks trying to apply it!

We were taught to say, "I feel," (whatever you feel or felt), "about" (whatever the situation is or was), "because," (the reason). For instance: "I feel angry about the time you told me a lie because I trusted you." Variations of this formula substituted the words, "when" or "if" or "about." Another example: "I feel sad when (or if), you are not open with me because I cannot know you." Then we would go around the room practicing. On the initial try, many parents would make a statement which included just one word which acted as a shield to their emotions. The word was "that." They would say, "I feel THAT you..." Instantly, this changed an expression of *feeling* into a statement of *opinion*! By doing this, a subtle shift occurs. If I say to you, "I feel THAT you are lying," the focus shifts from an expression of what I may be *feeling* to my labeling of how you are *behaving*.

It was difficult to grasp the difference. It took practice over a period of many weeks and sometimes months before some people could consistently eliminate "THAT." At first, when they lost their "that" shield, they would simply say, "I feel..." and then the stammering and stuttering and restless body language would take over.

Usually, the first true feeling word expressed was "uncomfortable," i.e. "I feel uncomfortable when asked to express my feelings."

I became aware with a few exceptions, almost every parent had difficulty with this simple exercise. What does this say about our early learning experiences? Our culture has evolved into one which greatly values rational, scientific thought. Unlike Eastern philosophies, we have separated ourselves into two distinct parts: mind and body. We have come to believe our minds are superior and our bodies are our more primitive, animal selves. We are mostly unconscious of this; yet, it affects us on every level. I could see the struggle in every parent who said, "I feel THAT." It was as though to allow the expression of *feeling* would be an evolutionary step backward! As a civilization, we have adopted the notion that it is better to think than to *feel*. We have related to feelings as though they should be expressed only in the bathroom along with other bodily wastes.

Truthfully, unexamined, unprocessed negative feelings *do* fit into this excremental category. By communicating clearly in the present, we must first rid ourselves of feelings from the past. Otherwise, we cannot speak directly to other people. We will be speaking only to our pain, finding ourselves stuck. We will unconsciously recreate the very negative situations we long to avoid. While we may consciously forget the actual situations in which our original emotional injuries occurred, our emotional responses to those situations are retained.

These emotional responses are carried around in our bodies like toxins. They erupt either physically or behaviorally, creating disease and chaos. Or, they remain with and suffocate our bodies and minds in depression. They destroy relationships. Many of the parents whose children were in treatment received an unexpected gift- they learned how to feel and how to comfortably and appropriately express these feelings. By constantly practicing this new way of emotional expression, it could become a habit. The new learners could further integrate this new learning by teaching others. Parent learners became parent trainers. Some parents approached this task with an almost missionary zeal!

As a result of our small group classes in expressing feelings, we became close to some of the other parents. Two of the single moms who lived in the area became our "buddies." We would return after the Friday night meetings to one mom's apartment. It was as though we had returned to junior high school and were having a "slumber party." We would stay up until 2AM, talking and laughing, sometimes crying together. We experienced the best healing substance known to humans- each other!

In the meantime, Burt was working *his* program. As in the case of most worthwhile efforts, progress was not steadily forward. He experienced set-backs in his attitude and motivation. His moods would swing. Initially, *our* mood would swing along with *his*. As we became stronger in our own program, we were able to tolerate these mood swings. Our healthy detachment gave him the room to find his way.

He was gradually given more and more responsibility. After four months, he was in the role of mentor to several young men who were beginning this demanding program. He had to deal with run-aways, physically chasing after and retrieving them. At first, this seemed exhausting and even dangerous. Yet, he probably did not endure any more physical abuse than is to be found every Saturday on football fields and hockey rinks throughout the United States. The stakes in *this* "game," however, were much higher.

Burt was experiencing the same joys and frustrations we experience as parents. He was investing his time and energy in other human beings, who, in the beginning, were *not* tuned into or grateful for what he was attempting to do for them. To some degree, we now shared the experience of parenting with him. This shared experience served to increase our bonding.

The exercises in responsibility helped to bring about a very high level of maturity in Burt. There is never any guarantee an addicted person won't relapse. It could be the next day or thirty years hence. It is always a possibility. That is why there is no such thing as a "former addict." Furthermore, there is no such thing as being a little bit addicted. Either you are or you are not.

People have two opposite views about addiction. On the one hand, they believe the addict is a lazy person who lacks will power. They believe he or she could stop using drugs if they wanted to badly enough. On the other hand, they view the addict as completely helpless. Expect nothing from such a person and you will not feel frustrated. Neither of these viewpoints is helpful. Both of them imply that the addict and the addiction are incapable of amelioration.

Several months after Burt returned home from the TC, he made this interesting observation concerning addiction: "Before awareness of his or her condition, one cannot expect an addict to take responsibility. After awareness, expect and insist upon the addict taking responsibility for his or her actions. Anything less is enabling and rescuing behavior." I would add to that: anything less is codependent behavior. It shows that the person engaged in enabling and rescuing needs treatment for the disease of codependency. One can receive help for the disease of codependency *whether or not* the addict is open to receiving help.

Once it has been established and accepted by oneself that one has the disease of addiction, *the responsibility for staying in recovery rests squarely with the addict.* There is a similar responsibility for those relating to the addict- family members and friends, the codependents. They must become aware of their responsibilities and *only* theirs, not those of the addict. *It is often more difficult for a codependent to stop enabling and rescuing behaviors than it is for the addict to stop using their drug of choice.*

For the addicted person, the best insurance against relapse is a heightened sense of responsibility. It is certainly a desirable character trait for everyone to have, but for an addicted person, it may be immediately life-saving. We could see the education in living which Burt was receiving through the TC was the best possible safeguard to his continued recovery.

Sometimes, he did not receive privileges which he had earned. This frustrated all of us, until we realized this is also a frequent phenomenon of "real life." He had better learn to deal with life's injustices without turning to the deceptive "comfort" of substances or addictive behaviors. Dan and I also needed to learn to do better with life's innate unfairness.

No system is perfect. For awhile, Dan and I actually believed the program had deliberately created unfair situations which we experienced. For instance, we submitted a request in writing within a set time limit asking for permission to take Burt with us to the airport so we might meet his brother who was flying in for a two hour lay-over. There was no reason not to grant the request; however, we received no answer. We were thus faced with the decision to act on our own. Relying on earlier information from the staff which stated "no answer doesn't mean you can just go," we gave up on the idea of the reunion. But, it hurt. Later we discovered the request had simply gotten lost.

At another point further along in the program, Burt had earned the right to attend AA meetings. It was not only a right, it was required by the staff as a responsibility. However, due to unusual circumstances, he had been placed as a mentor in a home where he never had any relief from his duties overseeing three or four other young men. For four months, he quietly managed the situation. Meanwhile, we submitted letters informing the staff of his plight and requesting an explanation which never came. For a time, we felt this, too, was an ingenious program which could plan such details in order to deliberately create frustration.

Then the staff began to criticize Burt for not attending AA meetings! We began to see it was *not* deliberate; the staff was clearly not communicating! Eventually, we did receive an apology; however, we became fully aware of the program's limitations. This knowledge was to be very important as we entered the final stage of Burt's treatment.

This program had five stages or phases. During the final phase of treatment, Burt was permitted to come home to live and return with us on weekends to participate in the program. We were elated. This is what we had worked for. Unlike many of the other young people in the TC, Burt had experienced being set-back only once in his entire recovery process. After he had earned the rite of "homecoming," he left the facility and came home on the bus. He did not use any drugs or commit any anti-social behaviors; he simply became frustrated and came home. We promptly took him back to the program. Strange as it may seem, he *thanked* us! I guess part of him knew he was not yet truly ready to make it on his own. He was a little older and more into his own recovery when he entered the program. Because of the extreme "either-or" way of perceiving reality which addictions programs generally have, he was never credited with having this advantage by the staff. They tended to err on the side of caution. We understood this. His progress through the program had been uncharacteristically swift.

Perhaps this is one of the reasons why they wanted him back. They *needed* him. He had become reliable and served as an excellent mentor. No system can be entirely separated from its own agenda no matter *how* effective it is!

As part of the final stage of treatment, the family takes a vacation together. This can be anything they want, depending on the amount of time and money available to them. At first, we planned a ski trip. We had a time-share available to us. However, Burt longed for a vacation in the sun. We found a bargain trip through an economy travel agency. As the snow melted in the north, we boarded a plane bound for Santo Domingo in the Dominican Republic. When the plane landed a few hours later, we were met by native bands and people serving a beverage in paper cups.

Shortly before departing, I had read a warning in a travel magazine by AA members concerning such a scenario. Suddenly, it flashed into my mind. Just as Burt picked up a paper cup, I yelled to him, "Wait!" Then I asked the young man serving the drink, "What's this?" He replied, "Ron y Coca Cola." I don't speak Spanish, but I knew "Ron" was not the man's name! How narrowly my son escaped drinking rum! This was a splendid lesson for Burt. It showed us all how cautious he would need to be all through life if he wished to avoid the danger of drinking alcohol.

The staff at the TC revealed their extreme "black and white" thinking. There was no middle ground. While this was frustrating, it was also understandable, given the thought processes of addicts.

They treated this incident as a total relapse! As far as they were concerned, Burt had drunk the rum!

They insisted he return to the program on a full-time basis. This created a crisis. Because he had been in treatment for a year and had been in jail four months before that, some major needed dental work had been postponed. He had impacted wisdom teeth. He needed them removed. They were creating an infection which was spreading throughout his body. He had already had the preoperative tests and an operating room had been reserved for surgery. The TC staff informed us this had to be canceled so he could return to treatment.

Burt discussed his decision to leave treatment without graduating. We felt confident at this point in his ability to deal well with life. We were also feeling disilusioned with some of the polarized thinking of the staff and administrators at the TC.

Burt phoned us and told us he had decided to leave treatment. This time, we supported him.

It was very traumatic for us because we could not say our "good-byes" to the parents. Some of them were permitted, even encouraged, to phone us with pleas for our return to treatment. Members of the staff called and wrote letters stating it was *impossible* for Burt to fully recover if we left treatment!. They meant well; however, they were too prejudiced in their own views to have any degree of objectivity. There seemed to be no room for individual differences in this treatment program. Obviously, nothing is perfect. Considering what they accomplished for us, however, this is a minor criticism.

We felt like outcasts from our own tribe! My regret for Dan and I is that, while Burt was ready to leave treatment, *we* could still have benefited from it. Dan was only just *beginning* to examine some of the issues from his family of origin; issues which had been affecting his entire adult life. No amount of counseling had penetrated *his* wall of denial. I could see possibilities with this program. Had we lived at a geographical location closer to the program, we may have continued in it. Some other parents had done this even after their children had left.

If a family leaves the program without completing it, the other families may not have contact with them as long as they remain in the program. Again, this is the peer pressure concept at work. Some of the families later reconnected with us which gave us great joy!

We came to feel almost privileged to have had a reason to be involved in the experience of the TC. We had struggled and learned and grown closer together. We had shared this journey with all its trials and triumphs with a great number of families. To do this was to be present, somehow, at the heart of humanity. It was astounding to realize the price of entry into this prized fellowship had been the pain of coping with our son's uncontrollable behavior! Who would have thought I would one day entertain the idea that Burt's addiction was a gift?

***

CHAPTER FIFTEEN

Wonderful things happen when one stops trying to control the uncontrollable. Possibilities present themselves! The opportunities for new learning include experiences which enrich your life and the lives of others.

As can be expected whenever new learning occurs, it brings with it the need in some way to pay tuition. This was the case one weekend in October, 1989. Dan and I traveled to Boston, Massachusetts to attend a parents' weekend. About six weeks before we had the opportunity to purchase a previously-owned, customized van at a very low price. We were frequently driving long distances and transporting young people, so we were thrilled with our new van.

Little did we know we were in for still another "learning experience!"

Necessary Steps : A Family's Journey

The parents' weekend was set up to duplicate the program which the kids experienced on a daily basis. There were strict rules which began the morning of the day we began. We were instructed not to converse with our mate or even have physical contact. We were to permitted to use the telephone. More rules would be added when the day's program began. We had stayed for the night at the home of some parents in the city. The van was parked in the neighborhood. It contained nearly all of Burt's clothing. We were transferring him to another house. There were several suitcases of our own clothing. We were leaving after this weekend to go on vacation. Also in the van was a brand new video camera. We had to leave our beloved thirteen year old Yorkshire Terrier, "Silver," in the van for the night. We didn't want to bring her into the house because a cat larger than "Silver" resided there!

Imagine our shock and confusion when we realized the locked van was not where we had parked it! It was *gone*. As we later discovered, it had become the victim of a "chop shop" auto theft ring! At the time, all we knew was- *our van was gone.*

All we could think of was "Silver!"

We promptly broke all the rules, talking to each other and phoning the police. Since nothing more could be done at the time, we proceeded to have another member of the TC drive us to the parents program. The TC member volunteered to call animal shelters in the area for us during the weekend in an attempt to find our pet.

As the weekend wore on, I became physically ill. All that mattered to me was the welfare of our pet. Yet, while it was difficult to concentrate on anything else, the demands of the program helped to divert my attention.

On Sunday evening at the conclusion of the program, we drove home in a rental car. Upon arrival, we listened to the calls on our answering machine and received great news: A "Yorkie" matching our dog's description had been found sitting on a curb in Roxbury, looking "like she just didn't belong there." She had been brought to Angel Animal Hospital in Boston. She was fine! We laughed, we cried, we hugged each other. We were jubilant! Even though we had just driven the four hours home, we immediately got into our second car and drove the four hours back for a soul-satisfying reunion with our pet. What was left of the van was found by the police three days later in Roxbury. It was declared a total loss!

Now, you may be asking yourself, what possibilities of learning anything could have occurred from *this* incident?

The following weekend, Dan and I were staying at the home of local host parents. We were relating what had happened to our van to a fine-looking young man from the TC. He was listening with rapt attention. "I know *exactly* how they got into your van," he enthused. Excitedly, he described, step-by-step how to break into and steal a locked van within minutes. "I should know," he concluded, "I don't know *how* many vans and cars I stole in order to support my drug habit-*too* many, I've lost count!"

Suddenly, an almost child-like look of total horror came over his handsome, young face. "Oh my God," he moaned and recoiled as though he had been kicked in the stomach, "I never, *ever* saw the other side. I've never seen anyone whose van was stolen. *I've never experienced what I did to them!*"

We have not been able to replace the van. It would be nice to do so. But, we know what is most important to us. The life of our son, the lives of other young people, and the quality of those lives matter most. The life of one small animal who needed to be with her family, and whose family needed to know what became of her, also mattered.

The rest is irrelevant.

***

CHAPTER SIXTEEN

March 6, 1993

I am writing this sitting in my kitchen where through large glass windows I can view the beautiful woods behind our house. The deck and ground are covered with two feet of snow and the hemlocks carry fresh powder on their emerald boughs. Earlier today, two huge red-headed woodpeckers were exploring the forest. They perched briefly on the trunk of one of the hemlocks. It was a breath-taking sight! As soon as I moved to grab my camera, they flew away. Some things cannot be caught. You must enjoy them in the moment and then let them go.

They reminded me of Burt and his friend who moved in November, to California. What we treasure most in life cannot be kept forever, except in the heart.

It has been over four years. Burt has remained "clean and sober." While his attitude has slipped at times in the initial stages of returning home, he has never "picked up" a drink or other drug. Thanks to the strong program which he received in the TC and later continued through the local Narcotics Anonymous (NA) fellowship, he has been able to recover his balance before reaching this point.

The first year after formal treatment ended, Burt financed himself through a semester at the local community college. He made the Dean's List! Naturally, we were proud. However, after half of the second semester was over, he decided this was not where he wanted to be at the moment. But, instead of simply failing to attend classes as he had in the past, he went individually to each instructor and explained the situation. It was *his* money and *his* time. By being honest with them, he was able to avoid bad grades which could hurt his grade point average in the future should he decide to return to college. This was certainly different behavior.

Burt did, however, have one large relapse in attitude. It helped Dan and I to realize how crucial our codependency program was for our *own* well-being.

After leaving college, Burt went to work repairing cars for his former buddy- the local drug-dealer. We were beside ourselves! It took all of ten seconds to feel ourselves back in that nauseating pit of despair! We immediately took ourselves to CoDA (Codependents Anonymous) and Alanon meetings.

Burt told us we were "being paranoid" when we expressed our feelings about his associating with people who were unhealthy influences. Fortunately, we realized it was not *our* responsibility to decide what was best for him.

Having stated our reasons, we then set our limits. Burt would, once again, have a choice: either he could choose another place to work, *or* he could choose another place to live. He had two weeks in which to decide.

"We're recycling," I thought to myself.

It is necessary to have faith in this process of "letting go" for it to work. *And work it did-* in a way I never could have foreseen.

During this anxious time, Burt was visiting a friend who had left the TC prematurely. The friend was scheduled to finish a prison term as a consequence of not completing treatment. He was in total rebellion. Burt stayed with him the entire night before he reported to prison.

The following morning at six o'clock, we were awakened by Burt excitedly barging into the house. "Mom, dad, wake up, wake up," he hollered. "I've *got* to talk with you." We thought at first he was using amphetamines- he was so agitated, speaking very rapidly. He told us while talking to his friend about all we had gone through in the program, he, himself, had relived his whole experience from addiction to and through recovery to the present time. "I don't know if I helped Ronnie," he burbled, "but it surely did *me* good to review the past! *I must be out of my mind*," he said. "What have I been thinking? *Of course* I can't associate with people who have any dealings with drugs!"

It was as though he had just found a lost piece of his brain! We were glad, but we had learned to have a very practical "wait and see" philosophy. Without us doing anything, he proceeded to do what he needed to do to take care of himself. He went to AA and NA meetings, found another job, and began to develop a solid relationship with his NA sponsor. This gratified us and reinforced our path of "hands off."

That June, we read in the local newspaper that Burt's drug-dealing friend had finally been caught, red-handed, dealing drugs in a "sting" operation. We were aware the police and other law-enforcement officers had been working toward this goal for several years! Burt was shaken to the core. He knew very well he would have been involved if he had continued along his earlier path.

Several months later, at the age of twenty three, his former buddy was sentenced to- from seven years to life- in the state penitentiary, for drug-related offenses. Recently, we learned two other young men, whom Burt knew from those awful days, are also living with the consequences of their actions. One of them was engaged in the manufacture of a street drug called "Ecstasy." He had enough chemicals to manufacture about one and one half million dollars of this "designer drug." He was sentenced "fifteen years to life." His younger brother received two years in prison for conspiring with him to market the junk!

In October that same year, we had to put our little dog, "Silver" down. She was suffering from cancer.

I knew it was time. Dan, Burt and I took care of this together. We shared our grief and our remembrances. Then, Burt announced he was going to move out and rent an apartment with some of the young men from the NA fellowship. It was time for him, too, to get on with his life. We were completely supportive. This time, we felt really good about this step.

During the following year, Burt experienced many friendships, including his first male-female relationship since recovery began. He was also able to serve in a leadership role in terms of sharing his experiences with other addicts who were just beginning their journeys. He spoke at various AA and NA meetings. He went back to the place of his enlightenment- the county jail. This time, he was the one coming in from the outside with a message of hope to lead a meeting of NA!

New Year's Eve, 1991, found all three of us at an NA Open meeting where we formally celebrated the third anniversary of Burt's beginning recovery. We were witnesses to a roomful of folks who praised our son and gave thanks for his strength and the power of his example in each of their lives.

I now understand the meaning of the term "natural high!"

Much has happened in the larger context of our family since Burt began recovery. Our son, Jon, Burt's older brother married and became the father of his own son. Dan took early retirement from his "drug of choice." He began the process of discovering other facets to his life. From time to time he relapses into living as an "activity junkie," and now and then, he informs me I have relapsed into telling him what is good for him.

As a couple we are far from perfect in our interactions. We have learned frequently we are not really listening to each other. We also learned that even when we *do* listen, we are not *hearing* each other. Many times one hears something that the other didn't mean. Prior life experiences certainly do condition the way words and behaviors are perceived! Just as Burt has done, we have learned the tools of recovery; it is up to us how we choose to use them- or not.

This passage in our lives greatly affected our entire family. Although Leanne and Jon were no longer living at home, Burt's behavior nevertheless impacted them. His actions and attitude had hurt them deeply. He had betrayed their trust, too. They wondered why this had happened in our family.

Leanne's immediate reaction was to handle her anxiety by turning to what she could control- her own life. Sometimes, it felt to us she was distancing herself, withdrawing from all of us. As she and her husband, Kyle, lived several hours away, there was little they could do. Yet, she and her family drove the distance to visit him when he was in jail. They even brought our granddaughter, then four months old, to the small, crowded visitor's room to see her Uncle Burt! Leanne used her pastoral privilege to arrange a private visit in the jail with her brother.

After Burt overcame his denial, he had to serve another one and one half month of his jail sentence. Pastor Leanne appealed to him at this time to write to her church youth group concerning his experiences and feelings. She was leading a youth workshop on adolescent drug use. I am sure his written account of past actions and their consequences was of great benefit for him to write and for them to read. It felt good to see negative experiences turned into something of positive use.

Jon, however, felt thoroughly disgusted. He was angry with his brother for the suffering his behavior had caused. For the first few months, he tried to understand. When Burt's actions continued to disappoint us, he announced, "I'm sorry, mom and dad, but I no longer have a brother." We had to take our sorrow over this to Alanon meetings. We could not control Jon's reactions anymore than we could control Burt's behavior. After Burt's turn-around, he had the most difficult task convincing his brother of his intentions for positive change. But, once assured, Jon was willing to drive for hours and inconvenience himself to be with and support his brother.

As a military physician and Marine flight surgeon, Doctor Jon now has more of an insider's view into the addictive process. He is quite good at spotting signs and symptoms of alcoholism and other chemical dependency. Furthermore, he better understands the disease of addiction from a systems perspective.

In May, Dan, Burt, and a treasured, long-time friend spent one magical month sailing from Alabama to North Carolina in Jon's thirty six foot Catalina sail boat. They experienced male-bonding in close quarters and encountered real danger at three a.m. as huge breakers nearly claimed the boat within sight of land! Temperaments were tested by spigots left running creating interior flooding! Pitted against the elements, both external and internal, the trio made a symbolic, as well as real, journey- a rite of passage. Only the three of them truly know the significance of this trip. For Dan and Burt, it seemed to represent the final bridging of a once large gap and the completion of a primordial paternal process.

Upon their return, it seemed a natural time for change. Burt had left home; but, he had been only five minutes away. He needed to know he could trust himself to be able to survive without us.

Burt and his friend had developed a dream of driving to California, joining some friends and finding work. They were setting out in the unknown. We knew we would miss them and he would miss us; yet, it seemed to be another growth step. We supported this dream. We feel closer to Burt now then we felt when he lived under the same roof. A feeling of gratitude and completion filled us even as we tearfully bade them farewell.

Recently, Dan received a letter from Burt. In it, he expressed these feelings:

"I went down to the beach alone, tonight, and it was beautiful. As I walked across the thick, brown sand, I could hear the hiss and thunderous rumble of the waves breaking. When I got close to the high tide line and stepped across all of the flotsam and driftwood, the sound of the breakers became almost deafening in the still night air....Memories of our seafaring journey came rushing back to me with stunning clarity. I am so very happy we had that time together. It is definitely something I will never forget and can easily call up in my mind's eye. I love you very much, dad, and it's near impossible to emphasize how much...thank you for my life. You know? The one you gave me and then helped me regain! I just wanted you to know how I feel..."

We will see him again, we know, and hold in our arms what is held, for now in our hearts. The visit, today, of the two, handsome, red-headed bird explorers with their strong wings is symbolic for me. Strong wings are built for flying- for carrying one's own weight in flight. I would not have it any other way!

To quote popular commentator and author, Paul Harvey, "...And now, for the rest of the story..."

It will take a lifetime.

END

THE TWELVE STEPS

1. We admitted we were powerless over:

   *alcohol
   *narcotics
   *person(s)
   *behavior(s)

2. Came to believe a Power greater than ourselves could restore us to sanity.

3. Made a decision to turn our will and our lives over to the care of a Higher Power as we understood HP.

4. Made a searching and fearless moral inventory of ourselves.

5. Admitted to a Higher Power, to ourselves, and to another human being the exact nature of our wrongs.

6. Were entirely ready to have a Higher Power remove all these defects of character.

7. Humbly asked our Higher Power to remove our shortcomings.

8. Made a list of all persons we had harmed, and became willing to make amends to them all.

9. Made direct amends to such people wherever possible, except when to do so would injure them or others.

10. Continued to take personal inventory and when we were wrong promptly admitted it.

11. Sought through power and meditation to improve our conscious contact with our Higher Power as we understood HP, praying only for knowledge

of our HP's will for us and the power to carry that out.

12. Having had a spiritual awakening as the result of these steps, we tried to carry this message to: *alcoholics, narcotics abusers, *codependents and control addicts, *behavioral compulsives

About The Author

Jane Barsumian is a musician, composer and writer. A former psychotherapist, she worked with adolescents and their families and developed an outpatient adolescent treatment program. Jane has written and led group programs in stress reduction and conducted parenting groups for various community organizations. She has also written poetry and original musical compositions.

Jane lives and teaches piano and violin in upstate New York where she is also a church organist/ minister of music. She was recently a recipient of a Woodstock Cycle grant with which she created and produced the musical drama: "Healing".

Printed in the United States
19419LVS00007B/2

Made in the USA
Monee, IL
26 January 2020